T0266745

# HEALING IS POSSIBLE

*New Hope for Chronic Fatigue,
Fibromyalgia, Persistent Pain,
and Other Chronic Illnesses*

## NEIL NATHAN, M.D.

Foreword by Jacob Teitelbaum, M.D.

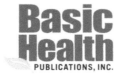

**Basic Health**
PUBLICATIONS, INC.

**AUTHOR'S DISCLAIMER:** This book is not intended to be used as a treatment manual, but rather as a starting point for understanding your illness and as a catalyst for initiating the next steps in your medical journey. As excited as I hope you will be to try the treatments described in this book, they each present a risk or danger to you or your family under certain circumstances. Therefore, do not embark on any treatment without the assistance of a medically trained, knowledgeable, and experienced professional who is familiar with the details of the testing and treatment programs described.

Throughout this book, with a few exceptions that are clearly noted, I have changed the names of the patients who have consented to have their case histories presented here. While this has been done to protect my patients' privacy, I have taken care to present their medical information as accurately as possible.

As medical information evolves, so does the work in progress that represents our life stories. By the time this book has gone to print, some of the details of medical information may have changed. What you read in this volume is the best, most accurate truth that I have access to at this time, subject to change at a moment's notice. I will do my utmost to stay at the cutting edge of those truths.

## Basic Health Publications, Inc.

www.basichealthpub.com

### Library of Congress Cataloging-in-Publication Data.

Healing is possible : new hope for chronic fatigue, fibromyalgia, persistent pain, and other chronic illnesses / Neil Nathan, M.D. ; foreword by Jacob Teitelbaum, M.D.
   pages cm
   Includes bibliographical references and index.
   ISBN 978-1-59120-308-7 (Pbk.)
   ISBN 978-1-68162-728-1 (Hardcover)
   1. Chronic diseases. 2. Nutritionally induced diseases. 3. Biochemical markers.
4. Chronically ill—Rehabilitation. I. Title.
   RC108.N377    2013
   616'.044—dc23

                                                            2013013621

Editor: Carol Killman Rosenberg • www.carolkillmanrosenberg.com
Typesetting/Book design: Gary A. Rosenberg • www.thebookcouple.com
Cover design: Mike Stromberg

# Contents

*I promised many, many years ago that if I ever wrote a book I would dedicate it to my beloved wife, Cheryl. I love the word* dedication. *It not only fulfills my promise, but it also describes our incredible relationship. She is my muse, inspiration, support, and nurturance, and without her, I strongly suspect that this book would not have come into being. Thank you, from the bottom, middle, and top of my heart.*

# Foreword

Although the rest of the planet is moving into the twenty-first century, most of our healthcare system is fixed firmly in a well out-of-date past. This book describes how having an open mind and an intellectual curiosity, combined with a compassionate heart, can turn a standard physician (an M.D.) into a cutting-edge holistic physician. This book can also teach you the tools that may help you reclaim your health—even when your standard physician mistakenly believes that "nothing that can be done."

## And Then Came Dr. Nathan . . .

A funny thing happens when a bright, well-educated physician sees treatments work that medically are not supposed to (for example, hypnosis, chiropractic, herbals). As Winston Churchill once said, "We often stumble over the truth. Fortunately, we usually manage to get up, brush ourselves off, and walk away quickly before any real harm is done."

But Dr. Nathan didn't walk away quickly enough.

In a world where most doctors only hear about the newest and most expensive (and most toxic) treatments, Neil Nathan has discovered that medicine has lost its way. Having found that numerous natural, safe, and inexpensive therapies work far better than prescriptions, he has dedicated his life to applying these discoveries for his patients' well-being. Though he tends to be easygoing, helping those patients who found their way to him was not enough. His caring and compassion have driven him to help as many as he can. So he decided to write this book.

## Hope

Are you frustrated with how medicine has become a cold assembly line? Are you losing hope that your doctor will ever truly understand you, or the impact your illness is having? Have you given up on finding a doctor who can actually help you?

Dr. Nathan's book shows you that there is hope in medicine and in a caring medical practice.

He starts where a doctor should—at the beginning: What are the simple and most critical nutrient and hormonal deficiencies? Magnesium deficiency, for example, can be presumed to be present in most Americans and causes unnecessary suffering and debility, as well as way too many premature deaths. The average American gets less than 300 mg of magnesium a day versus more than 600 mg in a standard Chinese diet, because of the magnesium losses in food processing. Encouraging magnesium supplementation—at a cost of a nickel a day—is not glamorous, but it could easily save your life. Dr. Nathan recognizes that hormonal deficiencies are also running rampant and are usually missed by our incredibly inaccurate lab testing. He then tells you what you need to know to take care of these problems. Having a doctor who recognizes and starts with the basics is a real gift!

From these basics, Dr. Nathan will take the reader into new worlds of ideas and inspirations that most physicians will never open their mind to—simply because those ideas are cheap and simple, and there is, therefore, no money in encouraging their being taught at the big pharmaceutical advertising orgies we call "scientific medical conferences."

What happens in Dr. Nathan's new world of natural healing therapies is no less than magical. Illnesses and problems that your physician said were incurable (and sometimes not even diagnosable) become clearly understood, and a path is laid out for you to reclaim your health!

Along the way, you will find that Dr. Nathan shares many personal stories about how the treatments he discusses have helped individual patients. Knowing Dr. Nathan well, I understand that he does this for a very simple reason. He takes his patients' and now his readers' well-being very personally.

I think you will enjoy reading this book. When you are done, you will enjoy reclaiming your health—and a life you love!

Love and Blessings,
Jacob Teitelbaum, M.D.
Author of iPhone application *"Natural Cures"* and the bestselling book *From Fatigued to Fantastic!*

# Acknowledgments

First, I would like to express my deepest thanks to Dr. James S. Baumlin, professor of English at Missouri State University. Jim took a fledgling writer/physician who had only completed a few chapters of a book, and encouraged, coaxed, prodded, and thoroughly supported that effort through its completion.

Next, I wish to express my profound gratitude to Casey D. White, who spent long days and nights converting my efforts into a completed manuscript and never seemed to tire of keeping me on track. Thanks, I needed that!

This book could not have come into being without the superb talents of Carol Rosenberg and the staff of Basic Health Publications. For this I am ever grateful.

I must thank, of course, my wonderful wife, Cheryl, for her constant support and encouragement, and also our three dogs, Kai, Jesse, and Joey, and our cat, Lucia, whose silent but palpable encouragement was noted and appreciated.

Without the dedication, commitment, and caring of my fabulous Springfield, Missouri, staff, Neva Dix and Kevin Joyce, this work would not be possible. The pursuit of healing requires a group effort, and I don't think I could have had a better team covering my back at all times.

Now that my family and I have moved to Northern California, I am part of a new team at Gordon Medical Associates, and I am grateful to Eric Gordon, M.D., my friend and colleague, as well as our associates, Wayne Anderson, N.D., P.A.; Alan McDaniel, M.D.; Annemieke Austin, M.D.; Mara Williams, F.N.P.; Julie Galvan, C.M.T.; and the entire staff for covering my front at all times too.

I am honored to have Jacob Teitelbaum, M.D., a pioneer in the treatment of fibromyalgia and chronic fatigue, comment on this new model of understanding illness in his foreword to this book. Jacob has been a wonderful support for me throughout this journey and his friendship is deeply appreciated.

Thanks, too, to my brother Gene Nathan, M.D., and Gene Shippen, M.D.; Ritchie Shoemaker, M.D.; Rich van Konynenburg, Ph.D.; and the entire Ratna Ling Fellowship, as well as Carolyn McMakin, D.C., and Len Ochs, Ph.D., for their support, inspiration, brilliance, insights, kindness, and most of all, their friendship.

And last, but never least, I wish to thank all my patients for their patience, hard work, and willingness to teach me everything they know. While medical science has many opinions, my patients carry the truth of their responses to our treatment efforts with them, and that is where learning really happens.

My heart overflows with gratitude to all of you.

# A Book of Hope

**W**elcome to my world! It is filled with hope, especially for those of you who have "fallen through the medical cracks." Let me explain what I mean by this.

If you live in constant pain or have fatigue so extreme that you can barely get through your day, this book is for you. If you have fibromyalgia or bowel problems and indigestion, or if you used to be mentally sharp but now can hardly remember why you have opened the refrigerator door, this book is for you, too. If you have numbness, tingling, and other odd or unexplained symptoms, this book is for you as well. If you have unexplained headaches, anxiety, depression, insomnia, or uncontrolled allergies, this book may be right up your alley.

Many of you have seen multiple health practitioners: doctors, chiropractors, naturopaths, massage therapists, physical therapists, and psychologists. Most of you have tried hard and spent a great deal of time, money, and effort to feel better or to get an explanation for your symptoms. Perhaps you've already surfed the Web, attempting to sift through a tremendous amount of information, only to become utterly confused by the contradictory opinions from site to site. If you've been lucky with your personal research, you might have found some things that have helped you to get a little bit better. Or perhaps you're just treading water. Or maybe you're slowly but steadily getting worse.

For the past twenty years, my practice has been composed almost entirely of people just like you. How that happened is a somewhat long story, and I'll tell that story in the first few chapters of this book. For now, however, I'd like to clarify the message that holds together not only this book but also my entire practice—the reason that I do what I do. Simply put, that message is *hope*.

To understand the concepts that create this hope, we first need to

understand what is behind the medical diagnoses and treatments that you
have already been offered—the ones that *aren't* working. Those concepts
and treatments are based on an old and somewhat simplistic idea that
each disease has one cause and therefore one specific treatment. This is
a delightful idea, and when it works, it makes medicine enjoyable to practice and yields wonderful results. Doctors' responses to many medical
conditions reflect this model: We diagnose strep throat with a throat culture and treat it with penicillin; we diagnose iron-deficiency anemia with
a blood test and treat it with iron; we diagnose blockage of the coronary
arteries with an arteriogram and treat it with a coronary balloon, stent,
or bypass surgery, depending on the specifics. This model of conventional
medicine has been in place for the last 150 years, and it is still taught in
medical schools and practiced by nearly all physicians.

The problem for many of you, unfortunately, is that most chronic illnesses are not caused by a single event or imbalance, but by a complex
interrelationship between multiple body systems. To treat them, consequently, requires a new model, one that embraces this complexity and
strives to understand and appreciate it. Understanding chronic fatigue,
for example, requires that we comprehend how your adrenal gland, thyroid gland, sex hormones, magnesium metabolism, and the digestive and
immune systems all intertwine. Identifying and fixing just one piece of
the problem (which would mean adhering to the old model) often leads
to temporary improvement, but the body just can't sustain that improvement. The remaining unidentified imbalances and deficiencies override
the temporary improvement and you go back to being fatigued. To heal
this fatigue requires some patience, a detailed understanding of the intricate relationship among all the possible causes, and a knowledge of how
these factors work together to create this fatigue in this person at this
exact moment in time. That is what this book is about.

In our current managed healthcare system, when only a quick visit
to the doctor's office is allotted, your primary care physician cannot
begin to address the magnificent complexity of your body. Under managed healthcare you are permitted brief, unsatisfying visits and are
quickly told after a short while that all of your symptoms are probably
psychological in origin. You emerge with the impression that because
your physician has a limited amount of time to work with you, he or
she doesn't quite know what to do about any of the symptoms you are

having. You would be right. Please understand that many, perhaps most, medical concerns are handled well by a managed health-care system. However, when things get complicated and require a great deal of time to review and sort through all of that information, a managed healthcare system falls short because it is not designed to do this.

After months or years of regular medical visits with no answers, no improvement, and no real treatment offered, who wouldn't become frightened and depressed? You've been wrestling with feeling truly awful for a long time, and then you are told that medical science has absolutely no explanation for your illness. This adds another dimension to your illness, but it's not the cause, and until we identify the cause(s) and treat them, you cannot get well.

From my medical perspective, the essence of healing is about diagnosis—finding out *why* you are not well. Without a clear diagnosis, we have no viable starting point from which we can evaluate your illness and treat it. In a nutshell, a clear diagnosis is crucial to beginning any treatment program; without it, we are just guessing. And how likely are we to be of help if we are just shooting in the dark?

Here's where I part ways from some of my colleagues in medicine. I am convinced that a more precise diagnosis is available for my patients using a new body of knowledge, sometimes referred to as *functional medicine,* which I will explain to you in this book. "Functional medicine" is a term that refers to a different way of evaluating and understanding the intricate, complex interplay of multiple systems in the body. This would include, for example, studying the balance of adrenal, thyroid, and sex hormones with neurotransmitters in an individual. Unfortunately, it appears that most physicians are not aware of this new information. But I have treated thousands of people using this new model of functional medicine, and I have seen wonderful successes. And that is why I am filled with hope.

My purpose in writing this book is to attempt to help you understand this new information that has been acquired over the past twenty years by a group of pioneering physicians. Each of them has recognized the limitations of the current medical model and has found useful, new fields of knowledge to expand upon that model. I am honored to be a part of that group of physicians and to have the opportunity to convey to you what we've been learning. These new fields provide us with much of the information we need to diagnose accurately your complex health imbalances and address their treatment in an organized manner.

In the first few chapters of this book, I describe my own personal journey of discovery and how I learned to put all of this new information together. I identify six major imbalances common to most of my long-suffering patients, and I call them the "Big Six." These are imbalances related to the adrenal gland, thyroid, sex hormones, magnesium, food allergies, and overgrowth of yeast and toxic bacteria in the intestinal tract. Each of these imbalances is featured in its own chapter and discussed in detail.

In the next group of chapters, I discuss some of the less common imbalances, which I call the "Little Six." These include imbalances related to heavy-metal toxicity (especially mercury); residual infections such as the Epstein-Barr virus (mononucleosis), Lyme disease, and mycoplasma infections; mold toxicity; amino acid deficiencies; hypoglycemia; and the newly identified central biochemical deficiencies of methylation chemistry. Although these imbalances are less common than the Big Six, they are nevertheless significant contributors to illness and often need to be addressed. Please understand that there are many more imbalances out there than the twelve emphasized in this book. It is not my intention to be encyclopedic in this discussion but rather to focus on what I believe to be the most practical common areas for evaluation and treatment. While I know that some of this information is somewhat technical, I will make every effort to explain these imbalances as clearly as possible so you can begin to understand the bigger picture of how all of these biochemical concepts interface with each other.

Later in the book, we will take a detailed look at the subject of pain so that we can learn how to be more specific and comprehensive in diagnosing and treating pain. This section will include a discussion of the fields of prolotherapy, a method of injecting the ligaments surrounding a joint in order to strengthen that joint, and osteopathic manipulation as examples of underappreciated treatments.

Finally, I will try to synthesize all of this information and discuss the emotional and spiritual components of illness. Why are we seeing such an explosion of these unusual illnesses at this time in history? Hopefully this book will bring us closer to some answers to that important question.

Welcome to a new vision of what is possible in the realms of healing.

CHAPTER 1

# Falling Through
# the Medical Cracks

## Or, How Did a Nice Boy Like You . . .

Although I am a physician, when people ask me what I do for a living, I find this a very difficult question to answer. Not because I don't know, but because what I actually do is not a part of conventional medical practice and it doesn't have a name. Over time, I started to describe it as treating patients who "fall through the medical cracks," and many people seem to understand this phrase. I also describe my practice as "complex medical problem solving." I think of myself as a sort of medical detective whose job is to discover the causes for the illnesses of those individuals who seek me out because they've not found what they needed elsewhere. The vast majority of these people have seen multiple physicians and other healthcare providers before they make it to my doorstep.

This field has evolved slowly over my forty-one years of medical practice. Initially, as a family physician I provided the full range of medical services: I delivered babies and took care of them afterward, performed some minor surgery, took my share of long shifts in the emergency room, and for many years was up all hours of the day and night providing the best medical care I could. Despite excellent training at both the University of Chicago School of Medicine and San Francisco General Hospital, I encountered many patients who I could not adequately help with my available knowledge and skills. I slowly realized that my education had not entirely prepared me for all of the difficult problems I saw day in and day out. So I began to look for answers elsewhere.

One of my first partners was a superb chiropractor, Stan Weisenberg, who, at a time when chiropractors and medical doctors did not typically associate, took the time to begin to teach me the rudiments of manipulative medicine. "Manipulative medicine" is simply a fancy phrase we use to describe the use of hands-on treatments to alleviate a wide variety of aches and pains. When I attempted my first "neck cracking" procedure, under his careful guidance, I was terrified. For those of you who have not experienced this, it involves a patient lying on his or her back, and the treating healthcare practitioner cradling the person's neck with both hands. In a carefully orchestrated but sudden motion, the person's neck is rapidly turned to the side, a maneuver often associated with a distinct cracking sound and/or sensation, which is intended to free up a vertebra that is "jammed" or stuck. This maneuver often relieves pain and improves joint mobility immediately. Over time, I began to appreciate the precision and palpatory skills necessary to both diagnose and treat musculoskeletal problems, and I developed a deep admiration for those engaged in this work. Later I studied with osteopathic physicians, chiropractors, massage therapists, and physical therapists, all of whom had somewhat different approaches—and all of these approaches were helpful for certain healthcare problems.

At about the same time, I ran into a situation that completely altered the way I looked at illness. While attending medical school in Chicago, I took an elective course in medical hypnosis merely because it sounded interesting. While fascinated, I didn't have the opportunity to see how this could be used in clinical practice and filed the information somewhere in the storage compartments of my mind. After completing my internship and a wonderful tour with the Indian Health Service in South Dakota, Oklahoma, and Alaska, I went to Mendocino, a small town in Northern California, to begin my medical practice. Within a few months of arriving in Mendocino, I was working in the emergency room one night when a woman entered with a severe asthma attack. I admitted her to our hospital and tried every known conventional treatment to try to improve her breathing. A consultant agreed we were doing everything possible to help her, but she continued to pant and gasp uncontrollably, and her labored respirations were exhausting her. Desperate to find something helpful, I pored through the books in our hospital library and found a single sentence in a medical textbook that casually suggested that hypnosis could sometimes be useful for treating bronchospasms (contractions of the bronchial muscles, which constrict the flow of air in the lungs).

My knowledge and experience of hypnosis at that time were rudimentary and crude, and I could hardly envision the process of this helplessly gasping woman following my finger as I slowly attempted to lead her into a state of relaxation. I explained to her what I wanted to do; with no other visible options, we resolved to try. In the most soothing voice I could muster up (considering the fact that I was almost as frightened by her condition as she was), I asked her to follow my finger as I slowly moved it back and forth in front of her eyes and gently led her through a basic relaxation exercise. To my astonishment, within fifteen minutes her spasms had calmed considerably, her wheezing and panting subsided, and she was breathing almost normally. I had not imagined that this could be possible. She continued to do extremely well and was able to leave the hospital the next day. I continued to work with her using hypnosis at my office, and as we explored the causes for this episode, she confessed that her breathing difficulties began when she learned that her son was going to marry a woman she did not approve of. As she began to process and adjust to this stressful situation, her health improved steadily.

Keep in mind that this was 1974, and nowhere in my medical training had it been suggested that intense stress could produce this sort of illness. The reality of this information was staring me in the face; here was a potentially invaluable tool, and I realized I had to learn more about how to work with it. I began to read everything I could get my hands on about hypnosis and discovered that it had a long tradition of successful treatment for a wide variety of medical conditions, including headaches, anxiety, depression, bed-wetting, and low back pain, among others. I began to explore its use whenever I ran into a medical situation where my customary tools were ineffective.

Several months later, a woman came into the office with severe rheumatoid arthritis and peptic ulcer disease. These were somewhat related, since the medications we use to treat rheumatoid arthritis (anti-inflammatory medications and steroids) often cause stomach irritation that directly leads to ulcers. By this time, I had learned how to use hypnosis to allow patients to discover the relationship between specific stressors and their illness. This woman recalled, under hypnosis, the exact moment when her illness began. She had owned a number of hair salons in Reno. She was working one day when an elegantly dressed woman came in with a doting family in tow. Her client had severe rheumatoid arthritis with classically deformed joints in her hands, and although she had great difficulty moving, her family tended to her every need as she received her salon treatment. My patient recalled feeling deeply, wistfully jealous of this woman, and in her financially successful but lonely life, wished that she, too, could be taken care of in this loving manner. Within a few weeks, she noted the onset of joint pain; within a year she had fully developed severe rheumatoid arthritis. She became disabled and had to sell her chain of salons. Eventually she moved to a small town just north of my medical practice, purchasing a small motel that she ran with the help of others. She had become increasingly disabled by the time she sought my help. Because her ulcers prevented her from taking the usual medications that we used to treat this disease, and with no other options known to me at that time, I offered the use of hypnosis to explore and treat her illness. She agreed.

Using my newly learned skills, she discovered fairly quickly how her illness had begun. But how could we treat it? As we explored her illness, it became obvious that she was holding on to a great deal of suppressed feelings that predated her illness. While she was hypnotized, I offered her the opportunity to allow herself to both feel and express those emotions; over several sessions, she wept and sobbed and raged. With this release of emotions, and again to my amazement, she began to improve. Not only did she improve, but her illness disappeared completely as well. All traces of rheumatoid arthritis were gone; her blood tests returned to normal; and, most astonishing, the joints of her hands returned to normal. She was able to stack cases of soda for her vending machines at the motel without difficulty, which would have been inconceivable previously. To give you an idea of the magnitude of this change, I read in my medical textbooks, repeatedly, that once the joints of the hands had deteriorated to this extent, healing was *impossible*. But there I was, looking at the impossible. There seemed to be a clear cause and effect here: The emotional events of this woman's life led directly to the development of an incapacitating physical disease. By understanding this process, we were able to reverse her disease.

Nowhere in my medical education had anyone suggested that this was possible.

That singular event raised the obvious questions: What else is possible? How did this healing happen? Can this method work for others with similar diseases? Can it work for others with different medical conditions? What other conditions are amenable to this approach? A whole new world had opened up for me, and I could not imagine leaving it unexplored.

Since rheumatoid arthritis is in the family of illnesses known as *autoimmune diseases,* I then offered my patients with the diagnoses of rheumatoid arthritis, lupus, and multiple sclerosis (MS) the option of exploring their illnesses in a similar fashion. Many took me up on it. Over several years, I treated more than a dozen individuals using this process of hypnosis to explore the cause and treatment of their illnesses, and half of them were healed; their laboratory work returned to normal, and all manifestations of the disease were gone. While it is known that autoimmune disease can occasionally go into spontaneous remission for no clear reason, my experience was way beyond occasional, and well beyond anything that we knew about these illnesses. I am not suggesting that all autoimmune illness is caused by stress, or that all autoimmune illness can be successfully treated by methods that focus on the effects of stressors on the body. However, I am clearly stating that the relationship between stress and autoimmune illness may be more important than we have appreciated. Perhaps more important for me was the realization that my medical training, as extensive as it was, had still limited my understanding of the possibilities of healing. There were more concepts and models of healing out there, which I had not explored, which might be valuable for some of my patients. Although I have emphasized here how hypnosis was one of those models, it just happened to be the one that started this journey and opened the door to further explorations.

This was the beginning of my understanding of what we now call the "mind-body" connection. One of the most important things I was learning was that it was not enough for my patients to recall their traumatic events. Unless they actually released the emotions that were being held in their tissues, healing didn't seem to occur. Even when they did, not everyone got well. Why not?

Another very different group of patients next came to my attention. The first of these was a young man, sixteen years old, who was referred to me from a group-care home in which he was residing. He'd had intractable, grand mal seizures (where the whole body shakes violently) for a number of years and was poorly controlled on his medication. He'd seen multiple neurologists and tried everything available; so again, I was left with hypnosis as the only tool I could think of to help him.

He was agreeable to exploring his seizures, and under hypnosis I asked him to relive the last few seizures, moment by moment. Every seizure seemed to be triggered by an intense feeling of either fear or rage. Again, I was surprised. I had always been led to understand that seizures were caused by random electrical discharges in the brain, but his did not seem to be random. What's more, this opened the possibility of a treatment: I reasoned that if this young man could control his fear or rage, before it precipitated a full-blown seizure, perhaps we could actually prevent them.

I taught this patient, under hypnosis, how to recognize and take seriously the intensity of his emotion, so that we could use a simple process to control it. When working with asthma patients previously, I had learned a technique in which the patient matches the intensity of their bronchospasm (the tightness in their chest) to the same tension level in their clenched fist. When they had precisely matched the tension level, and had control over it, the patient slowly, very slowly, simply opened their fist. As the tension in the fist dissipated, the spasm in the bronchial muscles came along for the ride and eased as well. I used this same concept with my patient's seizures. As he was now more aware of his emotions, I asked him to monitor them more closely. Whenever he felt he was becoming overly emotional, I suggested that he match the intensity of that emotion with the tension in his fist. When he felt that he had properly matched that emotional tension in his fist, he was to very, very slowly open his fist and let the tension/emotion go, until his hand was completely relaxed. This technique worked surprisingly well, and my young patient rapidly gained control over his seizures to the point that he was able to get off all medications and eliminate his seizures, all in less than a year.

My success with this patient prompted the referral of seven more youngsters with seizures. Again, when regressed under hypnosis to the moment of their last seizures, each reported intense fear or anger. Seizures were starting to look less and less like a random event and more and more like a predictable response to overwhelming emotion. Of these seizure patients, half were able to get off all medication, and the other half were able to better control their seizures on less medication.

Thinking I had just made a brand-new, wonderful discovery, I was amused to discover, years later, that Sigmund Freud had described this same process in 1908.

As excited as I was about these experiences, I was surprised that my colleagues weren't just as thrilled. In fact, most of them were uncomfortable hearing me talk about this. I'd expected from them the same kind of wonder or awe that I had felt, but instead I found doubt, cynicism, and mostly disinterest. That was the beginning of one of my most unexpected difficulties: how to interest my profession in listening to new information.

I found a willing ear in my chiropractic mentor, Stan Weisenberg, who not only seemed to understand, but also had been studying the effects of *emotional release therapy* on healing. He, in turn, introduced me to a wonderful Reichian therapist, Dr. Phil Curcurutto, who taught me more about emotional release in healing from a different perspective. Dr. Curcurutto had studied directly with Dr. Wilhelm Reich, a physician who had developed a technique using breathing coupled with certain movements and massage, to facilitate the release of emotions. Utilizing these techniques in my practice deepened my awareness and knowledge of the connection between emotion and illness. Dr. Curcurutto, in turn, had learned of another healing process, a technique called *osteopathic craniosacral manipulation* that was not available for study by chiropractors. At that time, this was only open to physicians, both osteopathic and allopathic, and to dentists. He urged me to pursue that knowledge.

This led to a trip to Colorado Springs in 1975 to study this new field. It is a branch of classical osteopathy, but at that time I had no idea what an osteopath was. I was simply going on my teacher's recommendation. So I wound up the only M.D. in a room of osteopathic physicians, studying an obscure branch of healing. This technique, which we'll discuss in more detail later (Chapter 17), requires an extremely light touch and an exquisite sense of palpation, neither of which I had at that time. Fortunately, the teaching faculty—perhaps the most incredible group of healers I had ever encountered—were very kind to me. They tried to lead me, step by step, to the perception of the *cranial rhythm* (minute, subtle, rhythmic movements in the brain and body tissues) and how to "manipulate" them. After three days of intense training in which I demonstrated no grasp of this process at all, Dr. Edna Lay took pity on me and guided my awareness into a clear perception of the subtle cranial motions, for which I will always be grateful. This experience profoundly changed my awareness of and ability to feel imbalances in the body and to help heal them. Learning these techniques required a deeper study of anatomy than I had received in my traditional medical education, so that my understanding of musculoskeletal problems improved dramatically. Perhaps most important was the deep feeling of satisfaction that came from using my own hands to help relieve pain. It is always a source of wonder that when I've finished working on someone's neck or back or shoulders, the pained look in his or her eyes is gone; there is a sense of peace or relaxation about the patient; and we have built a little more trust between us, which is a nice foundation for further healing.

As my understanding of these healing techniques began to grow, my model of illness began to expand in other directions as well. What I've described so far sounds like a nice integration of the emotional, spiritual, and structural components of healing. And it is. But there is more.

At one of the first meetings of the American Holistic Medical Association (the organization of holistic physicians, clinicians, and other healthcare providers founded in 1978), I was fortunate to meet Dr. Robert Anderson, who casually commented on how important it was to look for hidden food allergies in complicated patients. My respect for Dr. Anderson was such that I immediately began to evaluate patients for unsuspected food allergies and found this to be far more common than I had been taught in medical school. At about this time, Drs. Orian Truss and William Crook began to write about intestinal yeast (candida) infections as another major contributor to poor health, and this opened up another field for study and treatment. And by the mid-1980s, hypoglycemia (low blood sugar) emerged as another missing piece of this puzzle. It was fascinating, too, watching how conventional medicine declined to embrace this information. Traditional medical teaching simply denied that food allergies, intestinal yeast infections, and hypo-glycemia were valid fields of study, despite the fact that when patients were evaluated and treated for these conditions, they clearly improved.

I began to see a process of polarization: Medical practitioners were taking sides about how to look at those who presented to us with unexplained fatigue, fibromyalgia, headaches, depression, anxiety, and cognitive impairment. Conventional medicine continued to insist that these patients were psychologically impaired and had no physical component to their illness, while some of us were seeing something else entirely. Traditional physicians had been led to believe that stress, mostly psychological in nature, caused almost every symptom we couldn't explain in our patients, and for their anxiety or depression they needed either medication or counseling, or both. Those of us working in this new holistic arena were seeing these so-called psychological problems disappear entirely when the correct diet, the correct supplements, and the correct biochemical corrections were prescribed. It was becoming clear that the illnesses these people were manifesting weren't "in their heads," but in their body chemistry. It was increasingly apparent, therefore, that we had a lot more to learn about biochemistry. While the first "alternative" tool I utilized was quite helpful, adding these other modalities added immensely to treatment successes and changed my understanding about the causes of illness. My initial work suggested that "stress" was instrumental in the onset of most chronic illness, as revealed by my successes with hypnosis. Now I was learning that physical components of illness that were unknown to us at that time were emerging as just as important, perhaps more so. Clearly we could initiate treatment using many different approaches, and often coming from the physical arena was faster and less time consuming.

By the early 1990s, pioneering work by Dr. Norman Shealy and others had established that adrenal weakness (Chapter 3) and magnesium deficiency (Chapter 4) were major components of most chronic illness. Dr. Denis Wilson had begun to develop his concepts of thyroid deficiency with a unique approach (Chapter 5). We also learned a great deal about the overgrowth of toxic bacteria and yeast in the intestines as a cause of illness (Chapter 6). And newer laboratory testing enabled us to measure food allergies with far greater accuracy (Chapter 7). We began to realize that chronic infections played a significant role in weakening the body. Dr. Jay Goldstein had already described this phenomenon in the mid-1980s with his work on Epstein-Barr viral infections (EBV), but again, that work had been quickly dismissed by conventional medicine. We began to document that other viruses, along with EBV, may contribute to chronic illnesses, especially cytomegalovirus and HHV-6 (see Chapter 12). The whole family of persistent mycoplasma infections (including "walking pneumonia") and the explosion of Lyme disease emerged as whole fields of study (Chapter 12). By 1997, Dr. Ritchie Shoemaker from Pokemoke, Maryland, began to write about toxins from infective agents in our environment as contributing to this chronic illness picture, and eventually he expanded this concept to include mold toxins and Lyme toxins as treatable disease components (Chapter 11). Dr. Jacob Teitelbaum, from Annapolis, Maryland, outlined this new model in his groundbreaking book on fibromyalgia and chronic fatigue, *From Fatigued to Fantastic!*

We will go over all these ideas in much more detail, but the bigger picture, as it slowly emerged (so slowly as to go almost unnoticed at times), was that we were finding physical and biochemical deficiencies and imbalances as the root cause of our patients' suffering. When we correctly identified the chemical imbalances and treated them, often everything else got better too. People who had been told they would have to live with feeling depressed, anxious, and fatigued were frequently cured and had no further need for the medications that had been prescribed. We now had the beginnings of a whole new model for understanding chronic illness, which allowed us to help many people who had almost given up hope. That model continues to expand, and every year we acquire new information and tools to improve our abilities to assist in the healing process.

This growing body of information also helped me to understand that there was a whole world of healing out there, and that some of its techniques could help patients for whom my traditional medical skills were ineffective. Combining conventional medicine with this growing field of knowledge, which is now often called *holistic, alternative, complementary,* or *integrative medicine,* made a lot of sense. I could help significantly more people than ever before, and just as importantly, I had new ways, or models, of how to understand their individual illnesses.

Over time, I started to see more and more complicated patients.

While I still dealt with sore throats and colds, my time was increasingly taken up with using these new concepts and ideas I had learned to help individuals to heal when others had not been successful in treating them. As I solved certain problems, new patients came with even more complicated stories, and I needed more information to be able to help them. This evolved into an interesting ebb and flow: I would feel inadequate about my ability to solve a particular individual's problems with the information at my disposal, and so I would be motivated to search out new fields to study. I would bring this new information back into my practice, and it would help some of the more difficult patients get better. Then, just when I began to feel like I was really beginning to understand what I was doing, patients with even more complicated symptoms arrived at my doorstep, seeking treatment. Again feeling inadequate, I pushed forward to find yet more promising new fields to study.

I now have a long waiting list, and my staff and I have to work hard to prioritize our time so that we can take on the most difficult patients and refer those who are less ill to others. This book is written with these individuals in mind—I would like to share my experience and knowledge with others so that those who have "fallen through the medical cracks" will know that there is hope for themselves and their families on these pages. It is my hope that this book will provide a starting point and direction so that they can begin their journey of healing.

# CHAPTER 2

# Starting the Journey:
# The First Office Visit

## Looking for Dr. Right

Most of my patients have had a long history of unsatisfactory visits to a wide variety of healthcare providers. For many years, each time they make a new appointment, they are hopeful that their needs will finally be addressed and that they will receive the help that they so desperately need. When each new visit proves to be yet another disappointment, they become, understandably, jaded and defensive. Their medical histories have become so complicated that they rarely feel heard, and they invariably leave the visit with the clear sense that their new practitioner thinks their symptoms are primarily psychological. Once again, they are often offered another antidepressant and a referral for psychotherapy, which they have gamely tried in the past with little or no success.

By the time this person has reached my office, they have seen anywhere from five to forty practitioners. They have not yet given up hope, but neither can they work up a lot of enthusiasm for another interaction that they fear will duplicate those that preceded this one.

Before we launch into the meat of this book, I would like to offer some suggestions and thoughts about how to select a healthcare provider who might finally begin to meet your needs.

### WHAT I AM HOPING YOU WILL EXPERIENCE FROM MY OFFICE

One of my long-held fantasies—to which I still cling after forty-one years—is that I will be able to help every single person who walks into my office. I am not so naïve as to think this is possible, but it is with that intent that I walk into the examining room.

I hope that I will be able to manifest every one of the ten qualities that I have listed for the ideal practitioner and office visit. I hope that you will feel truly heard and understood. I hope that you will feel my compassion and caring, and that my store of knowledge and information will be sufficient to allow us to begin a new phase of your journey into health. I hope that I will be open enough to allow you to express yourself fully, even emotionally, and that at the end of our visit you will have the distinct feeling that there is, indeed, true hope that healing is now possible.

I hope that you will have a clear idea of what I am offering, and that this will enable you to have a clear idea of what you are willing to do on your part. We have to do this together. I need to honor your perceptions, and you need to know that my staff and I are doing our best. If we can start with this clarity, we can go a long way.

## Ten Qualities to Look for in a New Physician and Office Staff

1. Compassion

2. A sense of humor

3. Patience and a calm demeanor

4. In-depth knowledge of the field of medicine that pertains to your illness

5. A first office visit that is at least an hour long, preferably longer

6. A caring and competent office staff

7. Emotional awareness

8. Spiritual awareness

9. Sensitivity to the financial aspects of health care

10. Experience and communication skills

It is very important to all of us that we make you comfortable and convey the message that healing is possible. Central to this process is the building of trust between us. Actually, you have no reason to trust me. Since the majority of my new patients have been "through the mill" and spent a great deal of time and money getting frustrated, not feeling heard, and going nowhere, I realize that I have to work to create some kind of bond or working relationship that you have not experienced before. I do not take this for granted. Rather, I will review your information in enough detail that I can honestly offer you genuine hope that you *can* improve or heal.

Usually, your response to my suggestions over the first few months (based on your history and lab work) will convince you that healing is possible. Once that begins to occur, we have the first spark of trust, and I try to nurture that spark and build upon it. As improvement occurs, usually in fits and starts, we build slowly and carefully upon it, with the hope of each visit uncovering yet another puzzle piece that will allow us to understand your illness and treat it better. Sometimes, patients who are understandably motivated to move forward as soon as possible push me to do everything at once. As eager as I am to do this, long years of experience have taught me that this will usually lead to confusion about what is working and what is not, and then we have to go back to square one again and lose ground. I hate losing ground, since it may lead to a loss of trust and hope, both of which are essential to what we are trying to build. Together we go slowly, step by step, looking for the pieces of information that will move us in the direction of healing. This is a serious work in progress, and as long as we stay patient and focused, it is my experience that good things will happen most of the time.

I would like to emphasize here—and I will repeat this throughout the book—that *the central focus of each visit is to make a clear diagnosis*. We must identify with precision the cause(s) of your symptoms in order to treat those causes correctly. Otherwise, we are simply shooting in the dark. Now, if we shoot in the dark, we might get lucky, but you can't count on that. It is obviously a better strategy for us to know, with some clarity, what we are doing. Therefore, my approach to healing is all about diagnosis. This seems like such a simple concept, but I fear that this process has been lost in the current practice of medicine. To be more specific: It is not enough to know that you have Lyme disease. We need to know whether your Lyme disease is complicated by mold exposure, the presence of co-infections such as Bartonella or Babesia, and the presence of other infections such as Epstein-Barr virus, chlamydia pneumonia, or mycoplasma. Even that is not enough. We need to know whether these infections and exposures have weakened your adrenal glands, or thyroid glands, or depleted your magnesium levels and compromised your ability to remove the toxins that are produced by treating these infections. What I am referring to as "diagnosis" means a clear understanding of ALL of these possibilities, and more (which will be discussed throughout this book) and how they interact with one another to produce your illness.

Before you leave our office, I want you to understand how we are going to get the information we need to make this clear diagnosis. Toward the end of the first visit I will put together what I call a "smorgasbord." I will try to summarize my understanding of your medical problem in as much detail as possible, and lay out a wide variety of explanations and treatment choices. I will solicit your input in what you want to do, and in what order. It is very important to me that you leave my office after your first visit filled with hope. And that you leave after every follow-up visit the same way. I suspect that you haven't had that experience before, and I hope to undo the negativity you have received from previous healthcare providers, which adds another layer of mistrust that interferes with our relationship and your healing process.

To illustrate the doctor-patient process I've been discussing, I thought it might be best to have one of my patients describe her experience for you in her own words:

## KATHERINE'S STORY

"Doctors, doctors, everywhere, but not one that can truly help me get well. So many meds, so many office visits and hospital stays. Eleven admits to the hospital in twelve months. Period. And I am still not well. The feeling that I am on my own, that I am being misdiagnosed, going through the medical maze. Even feeling abandoned when a doctor or medical staff member is aloof, unkind, or impatient.

"That was then. I needed to find a doctor that realized that because all people are different, we might not be able to be treated in the same way. I looked for that doctor a long time, and found Dr. Nathan about twelve years ago.

"With much anxiety, I did not want to start all over again with another medical history and more medical reports. At times it takes hours.

"I made my appointment with Dr. Nathan and finally I am in the office. A very quiet room, with overstuffed sofas that may seat four. Not rows of 50 or more plastic and chrome hard chairs, and a room so crowded . . .

"As we walk into the outer office, Kevin is there to great us. A very congenial young man. (Anyone under fifty is a young man!) Both helpful and knowledgeable, with a light sense of humor to put you at ease. At most we wait ten minutes, not forty-five or more. We are ready for the treatment room, [and hear] Neva's 'come in' in a very quiet but lilting voice. I feel I must be in the right place. Neva has a real gift to draw blood and the set I.V.s. She has a very sensitive touch and is a truly capable assistant. We proceed to Dr. Nathan's room.

"Dr. Nathan is a self-assured man with deep penetrating eyes and a warm smile. I know now I am in the right place. Okay, finally!

"'So what's happening with you?' he asks, although by the time he asks that question, he has a good idea. You spend about 60 minutes with Dr. Nathan and understand what treatments you need to help get you well.

"Now I am thinking, That was easy. Ho! There are lifestyle changes to be made. Some will take many months, maybe the rest of my life. 'You try this until I see you again,' Dr. Nathan says. If that doesn't work, Dr. Nathan always offers alternative methods, perhaps several. Sometimes when I think it is all too much for me, I am reminded of the sign on the door: No whining!

"A very patient doctor, most times more of a teacher than a doctor, he encourages you to learn, think, and read. Dr. Nathan has suggested so many books for me to read over the years, I have started the Neil J. Nathan Library Branch 2.

"We all need to take responsibility for our own illness and understand what is needed to get better. Dr. Nathan can't do that for us. He's here to help. Healing has to come from within ourselves.

"Seeking knowledge, taking responsibility, finding the right doctor may keep us from falling through the cracks."

## THE UNWRITTEN CONTRACT

We don't talk about this much, if at all, but every time we interact with another human being, professionally, there is an unwritten contract. If we are not aware of this contract, then serious miscommunications may occur. Even if you are not aware of it, when you interact with a physician, you have an idea about how that visit will proceed and you have expectations of how you will be treated afterward. It is really important that we talk about this, or both of us may be disappointed. I can try to communicate to you what I can do: Essentially this part of the contract means that while I cannot promise to heal you, I *can* promise to do my very best to find answers. On your part, it is important that you respond to what I have said and make it clear how you wish to be treated and responded to. If this does not happen, we are opening the door to a frustrating experience for both of us.

Before our first visit, we try to set the tone for that visit. We start by letting you know that your first visit will be at least 90 minutes long. Hopefully this sends you the clear message that I intend to take plenty of time to get to know you and your full history and medical condition. You will not be rushed. You will have the time you need to tell your story, in detail, and I will listen, carefully, throughout.

We ask prospective clients to bring their medical records to us for review. We ask that they complete a detailed questionnaire. Our questionnaire asks many questions not normally covered in most medical offices. Some of these questions are specific for, and unique to, fibromyalgia, chronic fatigue, Lyme disease, and mold toxicity. You may realize, as you answer these questions, that we are truly interested in the details of your case. We routinely ask about your possible exposure to mold, tick bites, cat scratches or bites, and horses, all of which might lead us to explore possible causes of your illness that are not routinely evaluated in conventional medical practice. Before we have even scheduled your appointment, hopefully we have already asked you enough questions by phone and e-mail that we have determined we are clear that we do have something to offer you. So, we start by communicating to you that we care enough to get this information and digest it.

Toward the end of our visit, I always ask my patients if I have addressed their concerns. Have I answered their questions? Is my thinking and approach clear? Do they feel our encounter is meeting their needs? I then make certain to communicate to them that I cannot promise that I can help them, but I can promise that I will give them 100 percent of my best effort and energy to assist them in every way I can in the service of healing.

The promise of healing is not one I can make. This is my contract. I will do my best, and the patient will do their best, and that will have to be sufficient. There will be circumstances when our best is not very good, but that does not mean we aren't trying. As long as we understand that basic premise, we can get off on the right foot.

I first learned about "unwritten contracts" when I worked in both an emergency room and medical office. In the emergency room, the unwritten contract is that I will look only at what you are specifically concerned about and address only that. If you have other conditions, even ones that may be related, that's not part of the deal. When I tried to do more with my E.R. visits, I was surprised to discover that my patients were confused by those additional efforts on my part: Why are you talking to me about diet and exercise when I have a bladder infection? In the office, the contract is different: There we are more receptive to a comprehensive approach.

In my current work—in which I see very little acute illness and almost exclusively chronic conditions—part of the contract includes my clarifying what I will do over a long period of time. Since we are primarily *not* dealing with acute problems, those seeking my care need to know that I am not available at all hours of the day and night. If emergencies do occur, we have mechanisms in place to assist patients, but most of the medical care delivered will be during office hours.

The computer has profoundly changed the way in which we practice medicine. The phenomenon of instant messaging with text, tweet, and e-mail, among family, friends, and staff, implies that I, as a medical practitioner, will also be immediately available to every question, thought, and idea that you may have. Not so. When I am fully engaged in my day's work, I want to be absolutely focused on the person I am seeing. I am not willing to be interrupted (as many of my patients are with their cells phones and texts during visits), and view this as a rude and unreasonable intrusion into someone else's appointment. Part of our contract needs to include my idea of what being "reasonably" available to you means. A common source of irritation for both physician and client is that this notion of availability is not addressed.

## WHY IS IT SO DIFFICULT TO FIND A PHYSICIAN WHO CAN HELP ME?

The vast majority of patients who show up on my doorstep are bright, intelligent, talented, and successful individuals who are baffled by the way they have been treated by the many physicians they have seen prior to arriving at my office. For the past twenty years and more, most of these individuals have shared the same story: They have made appointment after appointment with what they assumed were the best physicians, best teaching hospitals, and the best clinics, and every time they return home from these visits dejected, disappointed, and frustrated. They do not feel that their medical story has been listened to or appreciated and they feel dismissed as somehow "less than" because their symptoms do not fall neatly into categories that conventional medicine readily recognizes. As time goes by, they admit that they find it harder and harder to even make a new appointment because they do not want to be disappointed again. I would like to devote this section of the chapter to attempting to explain this, in the hope that it will help patients to understand why their needs have not been met, and perhaps where they should be looking to obtain the medical help they need.

Albert Einstein has been quoted as saying that "insanity is doing the same thing over and over again and expecting different results." Perhaps in this context, "insanity" is too strong a word; perhaps "misguided" is more accurate here. The central problem here is that those unfortunate individuals who have acquired complex medical problems are putting themselves into the hands of a medical system that is not designed to understand or deal with complexity and doesn't have the time to try. Conventional medical practice, as we noted previously, was designed on the concept of making a single, clear diagnosis and treating that condition with known, effective methods. That's great. But what happens when there isn't a simple answer: For example, how about the patients who present to me with Lyme disease and its co-infections, along with viral components of infection and hormonal imbalances caused by those infections and toxicity caused by those infections? The current medical environment is simply not designed to deal with this. If you have been sick for a long time, you may need to find a practitioner who is comfortable in working with a new model, a new paradigm, which attempts to understand *all* of the complex components of that illness so that you can work toward healing.

One of the central theses of this book is that we are, indeed, beginning to understand some of this complexity, and that this provides real hope for healing. However, if you are going to find this hope, you may need to move outside the boundaries of where you have been traditionally looking for your medical care. Again, most of my patients are baffled as to why there exist different models and paradigms, and alas, I cannot fully answer that question. I would like to attempt to explain a few things about how this has come about.

When I've been a captive audience on a long plane flight, I have been fascinated by some of the articles that I read in the airline magazines. Often there are pages that herald the "Top Ten Neurosurgeons" or some other specialty physician in a particular region (which turns out, actually, to be an advertisement). Patients sometimes tell me that they have seen the "top" specialists in their area prior to arrival in my office. I wonder how those physicians have achieved that status. On what basis. Who decides?

I have practiced medicine for forty-one years, and no one has ever asked my opinion about the "best" physicians in any area that I have lived. People are taught to scrutinize the credentials of potential practitioners, as if that information will help them select their physicians properly. The public is under the impression that if their physician has graduated from a prestigious medical school—for example, Harvard—

and is board certified in a variety of specialties, he or she is a better physician. I do not think this is always true.

There is an old joke that goes: "What do you call the medical student who graduates last in his medical class?" Answer: "Doctor."

The medical profession has gone to great pains to convince us that selecting a board-certified physician will safeguard us from inferior care. The truth is that board certification primarily measures a doctor's ability to pass a multiple-choice test. Board certification does not in any way measure compassion, kindness, in-depth knowledge, or the ability to communicate complicated information and address the emotional components of illness.

I know no method of evaluation that can look, in a systematic manner, at the ten qualities you should look for in a doctor and find that doctor for you. Difficult as it may be, you will need to find such a practitioner on your own. Nor do I think it is possible to find anyone with *all* of the qualities you are seeking. No doctor is a perfect ten, so you must decide for yourself what qualities are most important to you and seek them out.

Why is it so difficult to find the right kind of doctor for you?

Some of the answers to this question may be found early in a physician's training program. We select our medical students from collegiate pre-med candidates based on how those individuals coped with rigorous course requirements that include biology, chemistry, math, and humanities. The emphasis here is on mastering difficult subject matter, such as calculus and physics, which have, from my perspective, no discernible connection to the practice of medicine. So we encourage those with an intellectual bent to enter the field and discourage those who are more interested in human interactions.

I learned a great deal about this process when I worked on the admissions committee of the University of Minnesota's Duluth medical school. As a practicing family physician who had worked in small towns, I thought that my background would be ideal in helping to select new medical students who would fulfill that mandate. The first thing I discovered was that half of the admissions committee was composed of basic scientists (Ph.D.'s) and the other half of doctors in active practice. This is typical, by the way, of all medical schools. The basic scientists were strongly biased toward only those with superb grades and

MCATs (Medical College Admission Tests) as worthy candidates for admission. Those with good grades and scores and a strong history of interest in working with people were not even considered as candidates for an interview. This made it difficult even to look at promising individuals with "people skills." As often happens in political processes, we had to make deals with the academics so that we could support the candidacy of those who we felt had great clinical promise. If we voted in *their* preferred applicants, they would vote in ours. So even before our prospective physicians get to medical school, we have selected out a large group of individuals who might make fabulous doctors. Instead, we have offered space in medical school to many who are intellectually gifted but whose people skills are lacking. We are off to the races.

Then, during the four years of medical studies, we systematically dehumanize these aspiring physicians by making them work and study for exceptionally long hours. We neglect their creative and spiritual needs. We then put them through three to six years of extensive postgraduate training. During that time, there are no rewards for nurturing that person's individuality. By the time they leave their training program, most students are a shell of their former self. It was painful for me to watch my classmates at the University of Chicago go from vibrant, caring, interesting human beings to burnt-out automatons who were able to spout long lists of medical syndromes but had lost much of their concern for the patients with whom they had contact. By the time residency had been completed, they just wanted to finish their day and go home and rest. The spirit of discovery, of learning, of seeking new information, had largely been replaced by a sense of being constantly overwhelmed.

This exhausted group of physicians then went to work in managed-care organizations, where they were essentially told what tests they could order and what diagnoses they could consider. They were too tired to notice that their practice of medicine, and their enthusiasm for what they did, had been severely compromised.

In my generation, the "best and the brightest" readily chose medicine as their career. As medicine has evolved into its current limited condition, many more of the most talented college students are choosing other options where they will have more freedom to be creative and helpful.

Is it any wonder that your needs are not being met?

## RESOURCES FOR FINDING A GOOD HEALTHCARE PRACTITIONER

The ten practitioner qualities listed on page 17 may be found in many healthcare providers. Several organizations specifically train physicians to understand the body of information that I provide in this book. I encourage you to visit their websites to learn more. The best known of these organizations are the following:

1. American Holistic Medical Association with the American Board of Holistic and Integrative Medicine (AHMA, ABHIM)

2. American College for Advancement in Medicine (ACAM)

3. American College for Environmental Medicine (ACEM)

4. Institute for Functional Medicine (IFM)

Word of mouth is still the most productive way of finding the kind of healthcare provider you are looking for. A glossy website is not a substitute for substance.

The Internet is a hit-or-miss proposition in this regard. Some websites are accurate and helpful; some reflect a single individual's beating his or her own drum. Some chat rooms may add to your knowledge and others may spin you off in the wrong direction. Alas, there is a tendency for disgruntled people to vent their feelings in this media; people that are more sanguine do not have the time or energy to do so. The Internet is a double-edged sword, and it is not always clear which way the blade is cutting.

In the next part of this book, we will begin our exploration of exactly which biochemical imbalances you may have and precisely what can be done about them. My nickname for this body of information is the "Big Six." This simply refers to the six most common imbalances that I have found to be most often overlooked in the evaluation of chronic illness. Therefore, they are the ones that should be attended to first. Although there will be some discussions of biochemistry in the upcoming material, I hope to explain this in a way that helps you begin to build a picture in your mind of how we put all this information together to create a healing plan.

# PART ONE

# The "Big Six" Imbalances

---

After I complete my initial history and physical evaluation for every new patient, the next step of our first visit is to sit down and talk about the most logical way for us to begin our evaluation and treatment program. Each person is unique, and each story contains the clues that direct our attention to the imbalances that are most likely to be specific to that individual. But, as you might suspect, after a while we begin to discern patterns that are common to many of our patients. After years of analyzing patient records, it became clear that some patterns, some testing, and some treatments were more frequently observed in patients than others were. So, over time, I evolved a somewhat simplified system to streamline the process of how to make a clear diagnosis; this includes which tests to order that will be the most helpful and which treatments to initiate to begin healing.

To save my patients both time and money, we start, naturally, with the most commonly noted patterns of deficiencies of nutrients and biochemical imbalances that are associated with chronic illnesses., Then we move on to the less common imbalances. This process is modified by attending to the details of my patient's story. For example, if symptoms began following a severe infection, we might move evaluation and treatment of viral infections to a higher priority on our diagnostic list. If symptoms began following a dental procedure, we would evaluate mercury toxicity sooner, rather than later.

In general, however, I find that the majority of my patients have a group of imbalances that I have come to call, for simplicity's sake, the Big Six. New patients seem to grasp this concept immediately, and for most of them, the Big Six is our starting point for evaluation and treatment.

The most common imbalance, by far, for my patients with complex, persistent illness, is adrenal deficiency. While there are several types of adrenal imbalance, an inability to make an adequate amount of DHEA (dehydroepiandrosterone), the main hormone made by the adrenal gland, is present in well over 90 percent of my patients, so this the first step for most of our evaluations.

The next most common deficiency, noted in 80 to 85 percent of my patients, is magnesium deficiency and this becomes the next area to evaluate. Thyroid deficiency is statistically the next most common, and this is followed in frequency by sex hormone deficiencies, food allergies, and imbalances in the ecology of the intestinal system.

The majority of my patients have not one but several of these imbalances, and we have found that fixing only one leads to temporary improvement only, followed by relapse. So I attempt to identify as many of these imbalances that are likely to apply to the person sitting before me and to treat all of them. The response to treatment tells us where we have been successful and what we still need to do.

In other words, if someone comes back to me after I have treated all of their imbalance issues and tells me they are 60 percent better, this means that we have figured out 60 percent of what's wrong with them and still have 40 percent more to clarify. Then we move on to the next most common imbalances, the Little Six, discussed in Part Two.

I have discovered that this method of first identifying the six most common health imbalances simplifies the process of wading through what can seem like an overwhelming number of possibilities, which allows us to streamline this complicated process. So, without further ado, let's get started.

CHAPTER 3

# Adrenal Deficiencies

---

## DHEA: The Most Useful Test
## You've Never Heard Of

When it comes to diagnosing, treating, and healing long-standing medical conditions, in my experience, the single most important and overlooked area to look at is the functioning of the adrenal glands. In virtually all chronic medical conditions, the ability of the adrenal glands to respond appropriately to stress diminishes progressively as the stress of having that condition persists. Before we launch into this discussion, let's briefly examine the basic functions of these glands.

The adrenal glands are two small cone-shaped organs. One sits perched atop each kidney. They are essentially the stress glands of the body and are primarily responsible for how the body responds to all of the stressors placed upon it. These glands do not distinguish between the actual causes of stress; so physical stressors, such as surgery, injury, childbirth, or chronic pain, are just as much a strain on the adrenal gland as emotional or spiritual stressors. For the body, stress simply means the need to respond to change—any change. Even positive changes, like a job promotion, starting a new and happy marriage, or winning the lottery, are experienced by the body as stressful, though our minds may be blissfully unaware of this. Events like these might feel wonderful, but they are nevertheless processed by the body as changes, and a change in any form represents stress. It becomes clear, then, that merely feeling bad, for any reason, on a daily basis is more than sufficient to overtax and deplete the adrenal glands over time. For those of you who have been struggling with your health for a long time, studying adrenal function is our most logical starting point to seek out imbalances.

To oversimplify a bit, the adrenal glands make three major types of hormones: dehydroepiandrosterone (DHEA), mineralocorticoids, and cortisol. Those hormones, in turn, make other hormones or affect how other hormones function. So these three hormones are especially important to the body's metabolism. Let's discuss these three hormones in detail.

## DEHYDROEPIANDROSTERONE (DHEA)

The largest amount of hormone produced by the adrenals is in the form of DHEA, which stands for dehydroepiandrosterone. The good news is that DHEA levels are relatively easy to measure with a simple, readily available blood test. And a measured deficiency of DHEA is even easier to treat—with pure supplements that you can buy from any natural food store.

From the outset of our discussion, I would like to emphasize that if I had only one lab test available to me to provide help for my chronically ill patients, that would be DHEA testing. It is, to my mind, the most useful test I have.

Let's talk about DHEA for a bit so that we can understand the nature and value of one of our most important natural hormones. DHEA is a precursor for a host of other hormones, the best-known including estrogen and testosterone. In order for us to remain in balance as we wrestle with stress, we have to produce a wide array of hormones that allow us to deal with stress properly. If we can't, we lose the ability to cope with stress adequately—not only psychologically, but also physically.

This would seem to be a tremendously important factor to consider by any physician evaluating chronic illness, but for reasons that I cannot understand, this information has not received much attention from the medical profession. It is not unusual for me to see patients who have been researching their symptoms, and many of them, without benefit of a medical degree, have come to realize that they are probably depleted in adrenal hormones. When they present this idea to their primary care providers, almost all report that this suggestion is dismissed.

When we measure these patients' DHEA levels, however, they are universally low, and our patients usually remark, "Ah, I'm not surprised." It is unusual for me to see a patient whose DHEA has been measured by his or her primary care physician. Why? I suspect that many physicians have come to believe that the only possible manifestation of adrenal deficiency is Addison's disease. This is a rare condition in which the adrenal glands have been permanently and severely damaged, and patients with Addison's will require adrenal hormone replacement for the rest of their lives, usually provided by specialists in endocrinology. Somehow, conventional medicine has yet to embrace the concept that the adrenal glands can be temporarily weakened—not permanently damaged—and can be successfully treated.

---

### Symptoms of DHEA Deficiency

Essentially, a deficiency of DHEA causes fatigue, fatigue, and more fatigue (to emphasize the point). What's more, it also creates a slew of other symptoms:

- Tiredness
- Exhaustion
- Cognitive impairment ("brain fog")
- Depression
- Decreased libido
- Recurrent infections
- Generalized sense of "I just don't feel like myself"

---

The bottom line here is that we need an adequate supply of DHEA to be able to function. When we began our discussion of the adrenal glands in this chapter, we focused on stress in all forms. As any stress persists, whether physical or emotional, the adrenal glands slowly lose their ability to keep up with those hormonal demands, and start to become depleted. In my experience, the most common deficiency in most chronic illness is this deficiency of DHEA. Well over 90 percent of my patients with fibromyalgia and chronic fatigue are deficient in this hormone, by measurement, often to a profound degree. In fact, since almost any chronic condition is clearly associated with significant stress, we find a deficiency of DHEA in almost all of our patients. Those patients who have been receiving significant doses of a synthetic cortisone like prednisone, on a regular basis, can be virtually guaranteed that their levels of DHEA will be extremely low, because those medications turn off and inhibit normal adrenal function.

Since the majority of my patients have been sick for quite some time before their initial visit to me, fatigue is a problem for almost every one of them. One of my usual questions at our first interview is: "Please rate your energy on a scale of zero to ten, where ten represents a full tank of gas, and zero means running on empty." If an individual answers "eight or nine," that's pretty normal. But if the response is "two or three," which is quite common, then I have a nice, almost quantitative estimate of their fatigue (which of course is subjective), and I can use that initial number as a baseline by which to measure their progress as we move along in treatment.

## Testing and Evaluating DHEA Levels

Measuring DHEA is easy. It can be measured in two different forms. One of them is unconjugated or "plain" DHEA and the other is DHEA-S, where the *S* stands for "sulfate." I prefer measuring the unconjugated form because I have found it to be the most accurate measurement, especially when I am following it with sequential testing. Other physicians prefer to measure DHEA-S, which is the storage form of the hormone. Either way, a simple blood test can be used to learn quickly from where we are starting.

Interpreting these tests, however, requires a little more work and a little more information. The normal values for DHEA from the laboratory I use are 130–980 (ng/dL) for women and 180–1,250 (ng/dL) for men. Clearly, these numbers represent a huge range, and many physicians are not aware that unlike other tests, the reason for this large spread is that these values are *age-based*. This means that 130 is a normal level for a ninety-year-old woman, while 980 would be normal for a teenage girl. The same is true for men: 180 is normal for a ninety-year-old and 1,250 would be normal for a teenager. Once we understand this relationship—the fact that the age of the person and her DHEA levels are directly correlated—we can extrapolate the test results, by age, to find out what the number means.

Let's say one of my fifty-year-old males has a level of 200. A quick glance at his lab report would suggest that this is a normal level (and the computer obligingly places it there). If these reports are reviewed without understanding this DHEA's age-based "normal," physicians may be lulled into thinking that this value of 200 was indeed normal. But it's not. According to the clearly established age-level relationship, a fifty-year-old man's DHEA levels should be about halfway between 180 and 1,250, or roughly 600–700. All of a sudden, that 200 value looks awfully low, which it is. In fact, it's almost a third of what it should be, and it is likely that providing DHEA supplementation will make a big difference for this individual in his healing process.

You can see from the wide "normal" values for DHEA that it is an excellent example of a hormone whose levels decline profoundly as we get older. Some researchers have suggested that, to a certain extent, aging may be reversed by keeping DHEA levels close to optimal, although what that level might be is not currently clear. This concept has led some people to call it the "fountain of youth hormone." I am not prepared to go that far, but I am certain that measuring and treating this hormone deficiency is an excellent first step in beginning to bring a weakened physiology back to a healthy and sustainable state.

## Treatment of DHEA Deficiency

Just as diagnosing DHEA deficiency is a relatively simple process, so too are treatment and supplementation. Pharmaceutical-grade (high quality) DHEA can be purchased from any natural food store, and it is usually taken orally, in capsule form, once a day, in the morning. It is also available in cream form, but I find it difficult to accurately dispense a cream, and the absorption of creams through the skin is somewhat variable and not as predictable as I would like. However, the dose we use depends on the measured level of the hormone. I strongly discourage those of you who suspect a deficiency of DHEA from treating yourself. As with any hormonal treatment, guidance from an experienced clinician is important. Some people want to take DHEA routinely without measuring its levels, and again I discourage this. DHEA *is* a hormone, admittedly a safer one than some others. But you don't want to be taking any hormone or substance if you don't know for sure your body needs it—when measuring it is so easy.

Sometimes when I use the word *hormone*, people immediately jump to the association with female hormones, like estrogen, and they lump all these hormones together in their minds. This assumption makes them very leery of taking anything "hormonal." It is important for us to realize that we have hundreds of hormones circulating through our body at all times, and the fears currently associated with taking synthetic estrogens (see Chapter 6) do not apply to all hormones equally. Compared to estrogen, DHEA is a very different hormone, and as you will see, it has very few side effects. It is safe enough that the FDA allows it to be sold without prescription in health food stores. But although DHEA is admittedly a much safer hormone than most, you still don't want to take any hormonal substance if you don't know with certainty that your body needs it.

So, while they are uncommon, a few minor side effects may occur from using DHEA. In my experience, about 5 to 10 percent of women (and sometimes men, but rarely) will break out in facial acne from its use, and if this happens the treatment must be discontinued or the dose decreased. Some women will also complain of increased facial hair. Also, because DHEA improves energy levels, if it is taken too late in the day it may interfere with sleep; therefore, I encourage the full dose always to be taken in the morning.

One serious caution: DHEA must not be taken by anyone who has been diagnosed with breast, ovarian, or prostate cancer. To a variable extent, DHEA is converted by the body into estrogen and testosterone, and tumors that are hormonally sensitive could potentially grow in the presence of DHEA. This information has unfortunately confused some people into thinking that DHEA may *cause* cancer. This is not the case; in fact, the opposite is true. Research indicates that DHEA deficiency weakens the immune system, and hence there is an increased tendency to recurrent infections. Therefore, it is more likely that in a patient with a measured low level of DHEA, taking a supplement will actually improve their immune function. Understanding the difference here is vital: DHEA affects only existing tumors and does not produce new ones.

Having said all of this about side effects, readers should understand that the vast majority of people can take DHEA without experiencing any of them. It has far fewer side effects than aspirin.

As I will repeat throughout this book, the single most important thing to look at is how each individual person responds to the treatment we are providing. If taking DHEA leads to improvement, it is useful. If not, we have to question its usefulness, even if blood test levels are low. Note that it takes two to six weeks to see clinical improvement once daily supplementation has started. If no improvement occurs, we may need to recheck the blood levels at six to eight weeks to be sure the hormone is being absorbed and utilized properly by the body. Once a person has responded well, she usually can discontinue taking DHEA after about a year and not need supplementation again.

My office has measured and treated more than 5,000 patients with DHEA deficiency over the past twenty years. The response to treatment is so gratifying that I cannot think of a single test that has been more useful in helping to heal all forms of chronic illness. Most people who test low for DHEA will indeed respond with improvements ranging from mild to dramatic, as illustrated by the client case stories. Hence, this little measurement really forms the cornerstone of the testing process and the beginning of our looking for treatable biochemical deficiencies that will begin the healing process.

## TRAVIS'S STORY

Travis was thirty-five years old when he came to see me after experiencing some unusual complications, stemming from what he thought was just a simple injury. He had jumped over a short fence and fallen awkwardly on a rock wall, landing on his left lower rib cage. He was sore for several days, but he didn't think much of it until a rather violent sneeze one week later sent him into paroxysms of pain. Later that night, he collapsed while getting up to go to the bathroom. Sweaty and unable to breathe, Travis was taken to the emergency room by ambulance, and there he collapsed again, suffering a brief loss of consciousness, rapid pulse, and low blood pressure. For a short time he was unable to breathe. His doctors thought this was probably caused by a pulmonary embolus (a blood clot in the pulmonary artery), and he was immediately admitted to the hospital and treated for the presumed embolus. All of this treatment was completely appropriate, even though testing proved inconclusive, which is not unusual for this condition.

Over the next several weeks, he developed swelling in both legs, and his doctors documented deep vein thromboses (blood clots) in both legs, with a greater number on the right side than his left. These were aggressively and properly treated with heparin, a blood-thinning medication, with eventual resolution of the blood clots. But then Travis started to develop swelling of the lymph nodes in his groin and a persistent soreness and occasional "catches" in the muscles of his chest wall. He underwent a biopsy of the lymph nodes to be sure that this was not cancer. It wasn't.

Since his original injury four months previously, he had become overwhelmingly fatigued. Prior to this injury, he had been an energetic young man who held down a full-time job and also worked extra-long hours doing landscaping work. He was proud of the fact that he had been able to work these long hours for many years with no loss in vitality. But now, for the first time in his life, he was barely able to manage his primary job. Actually, he had to take several months off and was now only able to work six hours a day. He was so frustrated and upset by his inability to function as he once had that he couldn't even think about doing his landscaping work. He had been so proud of his physical strength, and now it was gone. He was worried about this bizarre turn of events following a seemingly minor injury and was starting to think, What could happen to me next? Now, in addition to feeling physically weak, with steady pain across his lower left rib cage, he was frightened as well.

At his first visit with me, Travis was clearly confused and afraid. He could not imagine how he could have become so profoundly weakened in just a few months from this seemingly trivial injury. From my perspective, his physicians had done a good job of treating his initial injuries and their sequellae (the blood clots), but they had not taken the time to explain to Travis the logical sequence in which all of these events had occurred so that he could understand them. Since his fear was palpable, my first task was to clarify this sequence for him and his family. After I explained to him that the injury had set off a delayed blood clot—which in turn had made him dizzy and faint and required the hospital care he had received—and that the lymph nodes in his groin were just normal responses to the blood clots healing, Travis began to see this chain of events as less mysterious and less fearful. I then explained how these physical stressors to his body had weakened his adrenal glands and that by measuring his DHEA and treating it, he could likely recover his health.

When I measured Travis's DHEA, it turned out to be 160 ng/dL, with normal for his age being closer to 800. I started him on 50 mg of DHEA each morning and treated his jammed rib cage with osteopathic manipulation (see Chapter 17). Within two weeks he was back in the office with a smile on his face. He was back at work full-time again, and he was no longer collapsing on the couch after work. His rib cage pain was gone. He had resumed his extra landscaping work and was handling it well, and he was now feeling like himself again. He was astonished at the rapidity of this energetic turn around.

I was not as surprised as he was, because we have seen this response so frequently after administering needed DHEA that we have come to take it as a matter of course.

While Travis's recovery is clearly impressive and a bit atypical since it occurred faster than usual, it illustrates how important and valuable it is to look for DHEA deficiency.

## KAREN'S STORY

Karen was a forty-year-old woman who came to us several years ago with a long history of thyroid problems. Several years previously she had been diagnosed as having fibromyalgia and chronic fatigue. She noted that on a bad day she would lie in bed all day and move very little, and on a good day she would try to get up and do things, and that really exhausted her. "My body throbs and my muscles hurt all the time." When she woke up in the morning she said, "It is like I've been beaten with a baseball bat all night." It would usually take her until noon to get dressed and start moving. She reported, "I can't handle stress; it wipes me out." She was usually irritable. Routine blood testing, including thyroid tests, was normal. Antidepressants taken over a ten-year period were of little to no benefit. She described her energy level as between "zero and two" on a scale of zero to ten. Despite excessive sleep, she was completely unrefreshed when she awoke. She had been researching her own problem and decided she had Wilson's syndrome (which we will describe in Chapter 5).

We started by measuring Karen's DHEA level, which came back at 224 ng/dL. A normal level for her age would be about 600. Noting this measured deficiency of DHEA, we started her on 50 mg supplements of DHEA each morning. When I saw her for a follow-up consultation two months later, she reported that she was doing extremely well and estimated that she was almost "85 percent better." She had only minor joint pains now, which mostly occurred when she overworked herself. Her overall mood had improved dramatically. We elected to see if just continuing this treatment with no additional elements would be sufficient to produce complete resolution of her symptoms, and it was.

So Karen is yet another example of the remarkable improvement that is possible with the simple addition of DHEA. While most patients are quite a

---

### Symptoms of Mineralocorticoid Deficiency

- Exhaustion
- Fatigue
- Tiredness
- Dizziness or lightheadedness especially upon standing up (technically called *orthostatic hypotension*)

---

bit more complicated than Karen, it is most gratifying to see someone get her life back so quickly.

---

If patients do respond well to supplementation with DHEA, but not completely, we may have to look a little deeper into their adrenal function to determine if the problem is beyond a simple DHEA deficiency.

## MINERALOCORTICOIDS

A second hormonal function of the adrenal gland is its assistance in helping to regulate blood pressure. The adrenals make what are called *mineralocorticoids,* a group of hormones that help to raise the blood pressure when it is low. Most of us are aware that *high* blood pressure is not a good thing, but it is not as well known that *low* blood pressure isn't good for us either. In essence, your blood pressure is very similar to the water pressure in your home. If your water pressure is too low and you try to take a shower, the water will simply trickle out of the showerhead because there isn't enough pressure to push it out of the spout. Low blood pressure is just the same: you aren't pumping enough blood through your body to provide adequate circulation, and this can lead to fatigue and weakness.

A particular symptom that can tip us off to the presence of low blood pressure is that of dizziness or lightheadedness when standing up or changing position abruptly. This symptom can be formally diagnosed by a tilt-table testing procedure, originally described by researchers at Johns Hopkins in the mid-nineties. However, in my experience, it isn't necessary to do this expensive testing to confirm the diagnosis. When we see an individual with consistently low blood pressures, and those pressures drop even further on standing up, we can make a presumptive diagnosis and work with our patient empirically. This means that we can simply provide medication for the unusually low blood pressure, presuming the presence of a mineralocorticoid deficiency, and see how our patient responds. We have the choice of two medications that specifically improve mineralocorticoid production: Florinef and midodrine. Both of these are prescription drugs that can raise blood pressure if it has been lowered by mineralocorticoid deficiency. How each individual responds to this treatment is our key as to whether we're on the right path to healing.

When I mention this treatment to some patients, they are frightened by the possibility that this will raise their blood pressure to dangerous levels. I can assure you that this isn't possible. The most I've seen these medications elevate blood pressures is about ten points for both upper (systolic) and lower (diastolic) blood pressure readings. This means that a pressure of 90/60 won't go much higher than 100/70. However, that small rise in pressure may make all the difference in the world to a fatigued patient, and it certainly adds another dimension to our treatment. Please keep in mind that this does not mean that everyone with low blood pressures needs this type of treatment. In the majority of individuals with low blood pressures, those pressures are normal for that person. Only individuals with chronic fatigue and a tendency to get dizzy or lightheaded when they stand up suddenly should even consider the possibility of taking these medications, and again, only under medical supervision

When we do use these medications, it is rare to need them for more than a few months. It is almost as if the body has forgotten how to make the substances it needs properly, and by this gentle medicinal reminder—given for brief periods—the body gets back on track.

## CORTISOL

The third main form of adrenal deficiency is that of the hormone *cortisol,* which is essential to a wide variety of healthy functions. When cortisol is not made in adequate amounts by the body, especially in response to stress, we see fatigue, exhaustion, allergies, hirsutism (abnormal growth of hair), and a tendency to miscarriage for women who are pregnant. But, as I have been emphasizing throughout this chapter, cortisol regulates the ability of the body to deal with stress of any kind.

Some of the most extensive research in this area was done by William McK. Jefferies, M.D., whose many papers and books are summarized in his seminal book, *Safe Uses of Cortisol.* Dr. Jefferies emphasizes that there is a huge difference between small physiological doses of natural cortisol and large doses of synthetic cortisones, like prednisone. (A physiological dose of a hormone is the amount of hormone that the body would naturally manufacture if it were able to do so.) Please note the difference between the words *cortisol* and *cortisone.* Although these words are very similar, we are often talking about different substances. Both cortisol and cortisone are the natural hormones made by the adrenal glands. Confusion about these words comes about because we generally refer to the *synthetic* pharmaceuticals, namely prednisone, as "cortisone" also. Since most of my patients are aware of the toxic effects that result from long-term use of large doses of synthetic cortisone, they are often reluctant to even consider taking small doses of natural cortisol, until we explain the enormous differences between the natural and synthetic materials, and the dosages involved.

The essence of Dr. Jefferies' research is that tiny amounts of natural cortisol may be restorative to the body when we have clearly identified cortisol deficiency, as opposed to the large doses of synthetic cortisone that are traditionally used in a wide variety of medical conditions and carry a much greater risk of toxicity.

In treatment, we begin by measuring an individual's cortisol deficiency so that we know what we're looking at. The test we use is called a *cortrosyn stimulation test,* and it is a standard test used in endocrinology for exactly this purpose. Natural cortisol is produced while we sleep, in what is described as a circadian rhythm. Our blood levels of cortisol peak at about 8 AM and slowly drop throughout the day, in this natural cycle. Thus, it is standard for us to measure a patient's baseline cortisol at 8 AM and then provide an injection of cortrosyn, a pituitary stimulant that *should,* according to Dr. Jefferies, triple the baseline level of cortisone when we remeasure it exactly thirty minutes after our injection of cortroysn (if the adrenal gland is working properly). If the adrenal gland cannot respond appropriately to this natural stimulation, which mimics exactly how the adrenal gland *should* respond to a natural stressor, then we know we are dealing with a cortisol deficiency. Dr. Jefferies aptly named this condition *mild adrenal insufficiency* to distinguish it from the much more severe deficiency that we know as Addison's disease, mentioned earlier.

We can treat these mild cases of deficiency by providing small doses of cortisone acetate, also known as Cortef, or with hydrocortisone acetate, which is just a little bit stronger than Cortef. Dr. Jefferies has found that as long as we keep the dose of Cortef less than 40 mg daily, there are virtually no side effects, even with prolonged administration of this hormone for up to forty-five years. As this is a hormonal medication, it can only be provided by a physician, preferably one trained in its use.

Once again, the individual's response is the key. If a patient improves with cortisol treatment, with a significant decrease in fatigue, we have identified yet another component of his illness. If not, even with abnormally low laboratory testing levels, we must go back to the drawing board.

We, as medical professionals must become more attentive to how our patients respond to different treatments. The truth of the treatment is in its success, or lack thereof, for each individual patient.

The nice thing about using both the mineralocorticoid and natural cortisol treatments is that once patients have responded, they don't need to take these medications forever.

As mentioned previously, but worth repeating, the majority of patients who take mineralocorticoids find that after two to three months, they have restimulated their adrenals into better working order, and their blood pressure has normalized and stays that way. For those who take hydrocortisone, the adrenal system is back up and running usually after a year or two, and the medication can be discontinued forever. Recall that the same is true for DHEA: Most patients placed on it can discontinue it after taking it for about a year.

What we appear to be doing with this approach is restoring adrenal function back to normal. And that seems to be a really good thing for our fatigued and chronically ill patients as they start back on the road to health, as Carla's story so aptly demonstrates.

## CARLA'S STORY

Carla was forty-eight when she came to see me, hoping that I could help cure her pain. She was on a slew of medications and had become concerned about their possible long-term side effects. She also wanted to know why she stayed so tired and exhausted all the time. "I would like more spunk," she told me.

Carla reported that, except for some minor aches and pains, she had been well until six years previously, when she received a flu shot. Two days later she developed a severe pain radiating from her left shoulder, at the site of her vaccination, up into her neck and shoulder. After the initial onset of pain, she continued to have pain between her shoulder blades and across her lower back and hips. Some days were worse than others. She had seen multiple physicians and chiropractors and had been given many diagnoses, including fibromyalgia, osteoarthritis, a bulging disc in her neck, and osteoporosis. She rated her energy as "five" on a scale of zero to ten. If she expected to get any sleep she had to take Flexeril (a muscle relaxant), and if she expected to function at all, she needed to take various pain medications and anti-inflammatory medications.

I tested Carla's DHEA and discovered that she was at less than half of the normal amount for her age. Her initial measurement read 235ng/dL, but for her age it should have been about 500. So I started her on 25 mg of DHEA each morning. I discovered that she had low levels of estrogens and progesterone as well, so I provided her with bioidentical hormones (see Chapter 6). I also found overgrowth of the yeast Candida in a stool culture, which we treated (see Chapter 8).

On this healing regimen, Carla improved somewhat over a period of four months. In addition to these supplements and medications, I specifically treated her hip, back, neck, and shoulders with osteopathic manipulation and injections (see Chapter 17). As is typical for many of these people with long-standing chronic illness, Carla noted that she got a little bit better after each treatment we added. Her path to healing was to be constructed of small stepping-stones. At four months into treatment, she was better now by "thirty to forty percent" by her own estimate. But she was still not completely well.

As we dug deeper to find the missing pieces of Carla's puzzle, we realized that her blood pressures were consistently low, measuring 94/60 on two consecutive visits, and she did get dizzy sometimes when standing up too quickly. So I offered her a trial of Florinef, 0.1 mg each morning. At about that same time, I conducted a cortrosyn stimulation test on Carla, which showed a baseline level of cortisol of 14.7 mcg/dL. It increased to only 29.1 mcg/dL thirty minutes following her injection of cortrosyn. For her, an appropriate response to the cortrosyn should have reached triple the original 14.7 mcg/dL, or 44.1 mcg/dL, whereas we measured it at only 29.1. Over several months we slowly increased her dose of oral Cortef to a total of 30 mg daily. She noted significant improvement in her energy and well-being as we slowly increased her dose. Now she reported that she was an additional thirty percent better with the treatments using Cortef and Florinef. Her blood pressure came up to more normal levels, her dizziness cleared, and I was able to discontinue the Florinef after just three months. As we continued her treatment program she continued to improve and now considers herself "almost cured."

Carla's story is evidence that identifying and treating these adrenal deficiencies can lead to improvements, even in those who have been ill for years. Further improvements for Carla occurred when we discovered and treated her mold toxicity (see Chapter 11) and methylation imbalances (see Chapter 14), but those are stories that we will tell as this book unfolds.

While the chemistry behind these deficiencies may be complicated, the essence of it is actually quite simple: Stress depletes adrenal function. The good news is that we can identify, measure, and treat these adrenal imbalances to begin the process of healing.

## FURTHER READING

Jefferies, William McK. *Safe Uses of Cortisol*. Springfield, IL: Charles C. Thomas Publisher Ltd., 1996.

Shealy, C. Norman. *DHEA: The Youth and Health Hormone*. New Canaan, CT: Keats Publishing, Inc., 1996.

# CHAPTER 4

# Magnesium Deficiency

## The Little Mineral That Could

The second most common deficiency often missed in those who have chronic illnesses is magnesium deficiency. Most of us have heard a lot about calcium, especially with recent concerns about osteoporosis in women, but while calcium intake is stressed, magnesium gets little attention. Calcium and magnesium are a little like two sides of the same coin: It is vitally important that they be in balance within the body. All of the cells in our bodies are bathed in calcium and filled inside with magnesium. The body likes it that way—it has elaborate safeguards in place to make certain that magnesium stays inside its cells and that calcium stays outside. In simple terms, you might think of the aging process as the slow leakage of calcium into the cells, which make them more rigid and less responsive.

For reasons that have not yet been clarified, most chronic disease processes cause magnesium to leak out of the cells and to be eliminated from the body by the kidneys. I've found that in 90 percent of my chronic-pain patients and in 80 percent of my patients experiencing depression, chronic fatigue, and fibromyalgia, magnesium is depleted. In some, this depletion is mild; in others, profound.

### Symptoms of Magnesium Deficiency

Since magnesium is a critical mineral in all muscle and nerve functions, when our bodies are deficient in it, we experience fatigue, depression, malaise, muscle cramps and pain, and difficulties with focus, memory, and concentration. In addition, magnesium is a critical cofactor in hundreds of chemical reactions in the body. For example, the Krebs cycle, which is the major pathway by which we manufacture energy out of the food we eat, requires magnesium for this process to take place. Our ability to make key neurotransmitters such as dopamine and serotonin out of the raw amino acids tryptophan and tyrosine (see Chapter 13) requires magnesium. So when we have an insufficient amount of this little mineral, we may experience multiple symptoms and organ difficulties.

---

### Some of the Major Symptoms of Magnesium Deficiency

- Fatigue, exhaustion, tiredness
- Muscle cramps, spasm, and pain
- Muscle weakness
- Poor response to manual treatments (chiropractic, physical therapy, manipulation); treatments do not "hold" or last more than a few hours
- Depression
- Cardiac arrhythmias (irregular heartbeats or palpitations)
- Cognitive impairment (difficulty with focus, memory, or concentration)
- Insomnia

---

## Testing and Evaluating for Magnesium Deficiency

Given magnesium's importance, why don't more physicians measure magnesium levels and treat deficiencies? First, most physicians don't know *how* to measure it accurately. When magnesium is measured by most physicians, usually in alcoholics and cardiac patients who commonly exhibit magnesium deficiency, it is usually measured by a blood test. As mentioned, magnesium is typically found *inside* of cells and not in the bloodstream. Magnesium is so important to a well-functioning body that the body will do everything in its power to keep blood levels of magnesium at a constant level. If there is a deficiency, the body will pull magnesium out of its cells to keep magnesium blood levels normal. Thus, you could have a perfectly normal blood test result but still have very low magnesium levels *inside* your cells.

The gold standard for accurately measuring magnesium levels is called the *magnesium challenge test,* in which magnesium levels are measured in the urine before and after the administration of magnesium supplementation. This test is rather cumbersome to perform, and I have found that a much simpler test is just as accurate: the *intracellular measurement.* This is not a blood test, but a scraping of cells from under the tongue—a procedure my patients fondly call a "pap smear of the tongue." The scraped cells are placed on a special slide and sent to a lab where the levels of intracellular magnesium can be ascertained. I have personally found this to be the most accurate test for measuring this critical mineral, and the results are often abnormal, even when standard blood tests show otherwise. Therefore, it is far more useful in making our diagnosis. Another magnesium measure, called *a red blood cell magnesium test,* is also available, but I have found that, while better than a blood serum test, it still misses about half of those individuals with significantly low magnesium levels.

Normal levels for intracellular magnesium are defined as 33.9–41.9 mEq/L (milliequivalents per liter). A mild deficiency corresponds to 33.0–33.9 mEq/L; a moderate deficiency is 31.0–33.0 mEq/L; and a severe deficiency is lower than 31.0 mEq/L. Making these distinctions is important because when the body is running low on magnesium, it paradoxically loses the ability to properly absorb magnesium from the intestines. Logic would suggest that if you have a really low magnesium level by measurement, you could just take more by mouth to make up the difference. Sorry, but this strategy won't work—and I will tell you why.

## Treatment of Magnesium Deficiency

Our bodies have a limited capacity to absorb magnesium from the intestines. When that capacity is exceeded, we get the one symptom that too much magnesium produces: diarrhea. In fact, if you think about it, milk of magnesia and magnesium citrate, which are commonly used as laxatives, take advantage of that side effect. However, while useful for treating constipation (for brief periods of time), oral magnesium supplementation works on the bowel by increasing transit time, a fancy way of saying everything in your intestines moves through the system much faster. When this occurs, it doesn't allow the body enough time to digest and absorb food, nutrients, supplements, and minerals—they all move through the body too quickly. So simply taking lots of magnesium orally will not work to accommodate deficiency.

For severe or moderate deficiencies, therefore, we find it necessary to provide magnesium intravenously. Doing this gives the mineral the advantage of bypassing the intestines, going straight into the body, and providing a larger amount for the body than it would obtain by simply ingesting it. A series of these intravenous treatments is often profoundly helpful in people who are chronically ill. I use a version of what is called the Myers' cocktail, named after John Myers, the physician in Baltimore who invented it. This cocktail includes magnesium, calcium, and vitamins C and B12. The number of intravenous treatments provided depends on the level of magnesium depletion noted on our intracellular test. Sometimes, however, even in the face of normal tests, patients respond really well to these treatments. There are virtually no side effects of the intravenous magnesium. While the original Myers' cocktail was often given by "push," meaning it went right into the vein, I find it much gentler to give this infusion over forty-five minutes to an hour. If given too quickly, individuals may notice flushing or headache, which resolve quickly as the drip is slowed.

Should all chronically ill people take magnesium? Probably. Note, however, that all magnesium formulas are not created equal. Most magnesium that you buy over the counter is entirely or mostly composed of magnesium oxide because it is inexpensive to manufacture. Unfortunately, the oxide form of magnesium is not well absorbed by the body. Only 10 percent of the magnesium in this form is actually absorbed. For other forms of magnesium, particularly the chelated forms, up to 50 percent can be absorbed by the body. The word *chelate*, which we will discuss in more detail (see Chapter 19), in this context merely refers to the fact that the magnesium is bound to a large organic molecule that allows it to be absorbed much better in the intestinal tract. I prefer magnesium taurate, which is magnesium attached to taurine (an amino acid commonly depleted by stress), thus giving my patients two nutrients for the price of one. Some manufacturers have suggested that colloidal minerals (which are minerals that have been prepared as especially tiny particles) are even easier for the body to absorb, orally, but to my knowledge there is no evidence to substantiate that claim and I do not recommend it.

## JIM'S STORY

While I have promised the majority of my patients that their real names will not be used in these vignettes, in a few instances I've been given permission to provide the true name.

I have known my osteopathic mentor and friend, Jim Jealous, D.O., for more than thirty years. He has always seemed to me to be in robust health, as we have hiked and snowshoed over the White Mountains of New Hampshire where he taught. So it came as quite a surprise when he called me a number of years ago to describe his recent health changes. Under significant stress, he had developed heart palpitations with cardiac arrhythmias, accompanied by fatigue with insomnia, elevated blood pressure, and an overall sense of feeling poorly. He reported severe muscle spasms as he slept, especially when he assumed certain postures. When he called, he had just been released from his local hospital, and despite the doctors' best efforts, he was no better. These symptoms were completely new for Jim, and he was worried that with the use of the medications prescribed for him, he was not addressing the real causes of his symptoms. So he flew out to see me.

With a little testing, it became immediately clear that he was working with a profound magnesium deficiency, which we measured at 31.6 mEq/L (normal levels are 33.9–41.0 mEq/L). This had in turn caused significant calcium depletion as well. Jim's calcium level was 8.0 mg/dL (normal levels are 8.5–10.5 mg/dL). Amazingly, his physicians had not measured either of these mineral levels, despite his cardiac symptoms, which included atrial fibrillation and elevated blood pressure!

I provided Jim with intravenous magnesium, calcium, and manganese for several days in a row and made arrangements for him to continue this treatment when he returned home. However, he was delighted to report that after his first infusion he was able to sleep through the night for the first time in eight months. By the time he left our office, he was markedly better. Within just a few weeks, Jim's fatigue had lifted, along with his overall sense of poor health. His arrhythmias had virtually disappeared, and his blood pressure had come down to a much safer, controlled level. As he continued to receive magnesium treatments, he returned to his former state of excellent health.

Jim's story is an excellent example of how replacing a single vital nutrient can profoundly and rapidly improve someone's health.

## FURTHER READING

Gaby, Alan. "Intravenous Nutrient Therapy: The Myers' Cocktail." *Alternative Medicine Review* 7(5): 389–403, 2002.

*Intracellular Tissue Analysis.* Intracellular Diagnostics, Inc. http://www.exatest.com/. IntraCellular Diagnostics is the laboratory I use for most of my magnesium testing. The website provides an extensive bibliography of downloadable medical papers on magnesium deficiency.

Seelig, Mildred. "Review and Hypothesis: Might Patients with the Chronic Fatigue Syndrome Have Latent Tetany of Magnesium Deficiency?" *Journal of Chronic Fatigue Syndrome* 4(4), 1998.

# CHAPTER 5

# Thyroid Imbalances and Iodine Deficiency

## If It Looks Like a Duck, Quacks Like a Duck, and Waddles Like a Duck, It Just Might Be . . .

Another common imbalance often overlooked in people who are chronically ill is that of thyroid deficiency. This discussion will reflect another controversial concept in our understanding of the chemistry of chronic illness. Conventional medicine has traditionally acknowledged only one form of thyroid deficiency, technically referred to as *hypothyroidism* (the prefix *hypo* means *low*), and sometimes called an *underactive thyroid*.

This accepted form of thyroid deficiency reflects damage to the thyroid gland, resulting in the inability of the thyroid to produce sufficient hormone. This results in a condition and symptoms that are easily diagnosed through blood tests of thyroid levels and then treated with thyroid hormone replacement. All physicians would agree with this classic definition of thyroid deficiency.

However, there is a growing awareness among some physicians that this somewhat rigid definition of thyroid deficiency does not take into account another form of hypothyroidism, which is actually not uncommon. People often come to my office having researched their own symptoms and are convinced that their thyroid needs treatment, but they've been told on the basis of repeated thyroid blood tests that their thyroid is normal and cannot be a part of their illness. I often find that that diagnosis is incorrect, and that we need to evaluate and treat this gland in order to move the individual toward healing.

The thyroid gland is a butterfly-shaped organ that gently wraps around the front of your neck. On the inside, the gland is hard at work trying to balance your metabolism. Because the essence of thyroid function is about the regulation of metabolism, deficiencies in thyroid hormone levels naturally create a sluggish chemistry that affects every part of the body. It should not come as a surprise, therefore, that low levels of thyroid hormones are associated with a variety of symptoms.

---

### Symptoms of Low Thyroid Hormone Levels

- Fatigue, exhaustion
- Constipation
- Temperature dysregulation (low body temperature, always cold)
- Hair loss (especially the lateral third of the eyebrow)
- Dry skin
- Menstrual abnormalities
- Cognitive impairment (difficulties with focus, memory, concentration, and depression)

---

The key phrase here is *sluggish metabolism;* every chemical reaction in the body is slower. As I have mentioned, countless people who feel ill have read about this and believe that they might have a thyroid problem—often to be told by their physicians on the sole basis of blood tests that they do not. How can that be? The problem here, I believe, is that there are several types of thyroid deficiency, and the blood tests available to us as physicians only measure *one* of them.

## Wilson's Syndrome

I would like to emphasize that virtually all physicians agree that if the thyroid gland is clearly and permanently damaged by radiation, surgery, or autoimmune disease (the most common type being *Hashimoto's thyroiditis*), then standard blood tests will reflect this and show definitively who actually needs treatment. People diagnosed with this type of irreparable damage should receive thyroid hormone treatments, usually for their lifetime.

What all physicians do not agree upon is the existence of another form of thyroid deficiency, one that doesn't show up on blood tests but still reflects a genuine need for thyroid hormone replacement. This deficiency is sometimes referred to as *Wilson's syndrome,* which must be distinguished from a rare copper-excess condition called *Wilson's disease.* Research on Wilson's syndrome first received attention in the 1970s from the writings of Dr. Broda Barnes, who felt that patients with low body temperatures combined with many symptoms of thyroid deficiency clearly benefited from thyroid treatment. Unfortunately, Dr. Barnes's work fell mostly on deaf ears. By the late 1980s, however, Dr. Denis Wilson picked up Dr. Barnes's thread and refined his treatment with the use of a specially compounded long-acting thyroid medication. This form of thyroid deficiency evaluation and treatment now often carries Dr. Wilson's name.

Here is the theory behind Wilson's syndrome: Under certain conditions, the thyroid gland produces enough hormones so that all blood measurements are normal. However, on a cellular level, the body may not be able to utilize this hormone properly. Thus, the body actually behaves as if it is thyroid deficient, even though the blood tests might come back normal. We have learned a number of mechanisms by which this may happen, making the theory an increasingly more scientific concept. If a person comes to my office with fatigue, constipation, weight gain, brain fog, and low body temperatures, even if her thyroid level blood tests are normal, she may well need to take thyroid hormone to heal. But if routine blood tests cannot accurately diagnose Wilson's syndrome, then how can we diagnose it? Well, there are several ways to clarify things; the simplest is a trial of thyroid hormone administration, utilizing sustained-release T3 in incremental doses (which we will go over in more detail soon). If a person responds clinically to the use of this particular form of thyroid hormone, with clear improvement, they have Wilson's; if they don't respond, they don't have it. It's that simple.

Unfortunately, in my experience, it is the rare physician who is willing to provide thyroid hormone treatment on a trial basis. I don't know why. This is not a dangerous treatment. Having provided this on a trial basis to 4,000 to 5,000 patients, I am convinced of its safety and efficacy. In all this time, we have had only rare and minor side effects, such as headache, palpitations, and insomnia, with no reactions of significance.

Part of the difficulty in finding a physician willing to try this is that conventional practitioners, especially endocrinologists, have already dismissed this concept as bogus, without actually trying it. I am aware that it is a rare endocrinologist in any area of the country in which I have practiced who would not dismiss this concept as being unscientific and unfounded. I am not aware that a single one of them has tried this on a single patient, which would make that dismissal just as unscientific. I readily admit that before I tried this form of treatment, I was also skeptical. But the immediate and profound number of success stories was overwhelming to the point that the truth became clear: This is a very valid, very useful concept and treatment.

I am certain that thousands of individuals with treatable thyroid problems are missed every year by our profession and go untreated. And because they are untreated, they continue to suffer, needlessly. Let's look deeper into why this is the case by examining just how the thyroid works.

## Thyroid Function

The thyroid gland makes two hormones, triiodothyronine and tetra-iodothyronine, nicknamed T3 and T4 respectively. The 3 and 4 refer to the number of iodine atoms in the molecules. T3 is considered the active hormone, meaning it's the one that does all the work for us. T4 must be converted into T3 in order to be effective. This is where the problem starts.

Under a variety of stressors, the body may lose its ability to convert T4 into T3. This means that while blood tests may indicate that an individual has sufficient amounts of hormones present, the body unfortunately cannot *convert* those hormones, on a cellular level, from T4 into the T3 it needs. Thus, for all intents and purposes, such individuals behave physiologically as if they are lacking T3 on a cellular level. Therefore, they truly *are* deficient in the thyroid hormone they require. Another important consideration is that both thyroid and estrogen hormones are transported through the body by the same carrier protein. This means that imbalances in estrogen hormones can, and do, affect the amount of thyroid hormone *available* to the body. The kinds of stressors that can create this imbalance, which Dr. Wilson refers to as "resetting the thyroid thermostat," include both physical stressors such as major surgery, severe infections, and childbirth, as well as intense emotional stressors. Remember, from the body's perspective, stress is stress. Once the thyroid mechanism has been disturbed, it may stay that way until it's treated.

Dr. Wilson was also aware that an often neglected and rarely measured thyroid hormone called *reverse T3* (also called rT3) has a profound impact on thyroid levels and body chemistry. Reverse T3 is a byproduct of the conversion of T4 to T3. But the more difficulty an individual has in effectively converting T4 to T3, the more reverse T3 builds up in their system and further blocks the conversion of T4 to T3. This becomes a vicious spiral, making it harder and harder for the body to receive the T3 it needs. This explains why some people seem to need more and more thyroid hormone (almost always given solely as T4), and why despite taking larger and larger doses they feel worse. What is happening is that they need a *different* thyroid formulation—T3, *not* T4, in order to meet their body's needs and to start lowering the elevated reverse T3 levels back to normal so that their system can function optimally again. Testing for elevated reverse T3 levels is another tool that allows for some scientific precision in the complicated process of treating thyroid deficiencies.

## Treatment of Thyroid Deficiencies

Since the problem with thyroid deficiency is T3 production, the usual thyroidal treatment of T4, in the form of Synthroid or Levothyroxin, can be seen from this discussion as neither logical nor optimally effective. The treatment administered should instead be a form of the T3 hormone.

Cytomel, a medication that has been available for years, is a synthetic form of the T3 hormone, and it is commonly prescribed. But it doesn't last very long in the body when provided in its usual form, which is a single dose of non-sustained release T3. To make things even more complicated, patients differ significantly when it comes to how quickly their bodies can metabolize Cytomel. Some patients need to take it every four hours to keep a decent level of hormone in their system, while others can take it every eight to twelve hours. Dr. Wilson recognized this difficulty during his research, so he got a compounding pharmacy to create a sustained-release T3 product—long-acting T3 (LA T3)—that would slowly and steadily release the T3 into the body over a twelve-hour period. LA T3 must be produced by a pharmacy that is knowledgeable and capable of compounding it (not your standard pharmacy). *Compounding pharmacies* are staffed by pharmacists who have received additional training to be able to prepare specially compounded products. and those products are available by prescription from any licensed physician. Patients being treated with T4 medication who do not experience significant improvement may benefit from switching to long-acting T3.

The important thing to remember is that even when your routine blood tests seem completely normal in regard to thyroid function, you can still experience low body temperature, fatigue, constipation, weakness, and changes in hair texture. If you do, you might be a suitable candidate for a trial treatment of LA T3. How can you tell if you have a low body temperature, short of just measuring it a few times? Well, you might have to do a little bit of math. I recommend that my patients take their temperature four times per day, for at least a week, and then calculate the average of those numbers. (An old-fashioned glass thermometer—if you can find and read one—provides a more accurate temperature.) Unless the temperature average is 97.8 degrees or less, it is unlikely that the patient has Wilson's syndrome. Additionally, we can measure blood levels of reverse T3 and compare those levels with total T3. My colleague and friend Dr. Alan McDaniel has demonstrated that those individuals with a total T3 to reverse T3 ratio of less than 10 are also candidates for this treatment with LA T3.

When patients come into my office and are already on T4 treatment, I wean them off it for a week and then begin a new protocol. For those who have never taken thyroid medication, or for those we are switching from T4, I start by having the patient take tiny doses of LA T3 twice a day, and then slowly increase the dose every three days. During this time, we carefully monitor both physical symptoms and temperature.

When we reach the correct dose, patients usually respond immediately. If a patient truly has Wilson's syndrome, there will be an obvious, often dramatic, improvement when we reach the optimal dosage that balances his or her chemistry. This will be demonstrated as a significant improvement in symptoms and a corresponding rise in body temperature. Usually my patients can put an actual value on their response to treatment, and I've had them report anywhere from a 20 to 80 percent improvement in overall feelings of well-being and good health. Since patients are so biochemically different from one another, the dose required (and hence the number of dosage increases attempted by the patient) will vary considerably. Please understand that I am oversimplifying a more complicated procedure for purposes of discussion here; this treatment should not be attempted without professional and expert guidance.

Now here's the best part: Once patients have responded to a specific dosage of thyroid medication, they can usually take that dosage for three to six months, be weaned from it, and then never need thyroid treatment again. If they are already on thyroid treatment, they often will need a lower dosage and will feel much better following this treatment. Unless the thyroid gland has already been permanently damaged, this is not a lifetime treatment. This particular treatment is a rebalancing program; once completed, the body usually remains in balance. On rare occasions I have seen patients relapse after intense stress brings the deficiency back. However, I would estimate that 70 percent of the patients I treat respond beautifully, which makes this a much more common deficiency than most physicians suspect.

As I reiterate throughout this book, the proof of this concept lies not in theory, but in patient response. The only way doctors can make this diagnosis is to *try* the treatment. How a human being responds to treatment is the truth for that particular patient. Be aware, also, that there are other approaches for treating the thyroid gland, most notably Armour thyroid, which is a combination of T3 and T4. However, in my experience, the LA T3 is much more effective in this regard.

## TANYA'S STORY

Thirty-nine-year-old Tanya came to my office in June of 2008 with complaints of fatigue, a constant headache, a generalized achy feeling all over her body, and some degree of depression. She had experienced fatigue even as a teenager, but as a teacher and a mother, she couldn't live that way. She told me that if she could, if she were allowed to, she would lie in bed all day. Starting with her early history of fatigue, she got significantly worse after the birth of her first child. She was given Prozac at that time, which helped a little, and she was told at various times that her thyroid was just sluggish. Modest amounts of Synthroid were of minimal benefit to her. After the birth of her second child, six years before she came to me, Tanya went downhill again. She had recently undergone a hysterectomy and she made it perfectly clear to me that she was having problems: "I am a raging bitch."

I began by measuring Tanya's DHEA level, and it was quite low at only 161 ng/dL (normal for her age is about 750 ng/dL). I started her on 50 mg of DHEA each morning, and put her back on a small dosage of Prozac. By her second visit, six weeks later, she was only a little better. Because her problems were clearly not stemming from just her DHEA deficiency, I asked Tanya to get an average measurement of her body temperature. It averaged 97.7 degrees, almost a full degree under the normal temperature. Along with her other symptoms, this low average temperature made Tanya an excellent candidate to try a course of LA T3 as a component of what I presumed to be Wilson's syndrome. At the second visit, after realizing that DHEA was not her only deficiency, I put her on the LA T3 protocol. When she reached a dose of 45 mcg of that compound every twelve hours, she noted immediate improvement, and five weeks later she reported that she was "better in every way."

Tanya now gets up each morning motivated and energetic, and she was able to move her entire classroom at the start of the school year without getting exhausted. "I can really tell a difference," she told me. She rated her improvement from the time we started the treatment at 80 percent. The enhancement in her overall attitude and demeanor was dramatic. "I'm actually happy now," she said. "And I'm not glued to the couch all day anymore." Her headaches are virtually gone.

We are looking at the relief of years of fatigue, depression, and headaches, after only five weeks on this method of thyroid treatment.

While most of the case studies in this book are rather complicated, here is a nice example of how quickly a simple intervention of LA T3 can sometimes work wonders.

## ELLIE'S STORY

Ellie, forty-six years old, was referred to us by some of her coworkers who were also patients of ours. Her primary concern was fatigue, and she rated her energy level as three on a scale of zero to ten. She also reported a severe abdominal pain that had begun just recently. We were able to address the abdominal pain with methods that we discuss in Chapters 6 and 7, but the fatigue was a different animal altogether.

I noted that she had normal thyroid blood tests, but that her temperatures averaged 97.6 degrees. So I offered her a trial of LA T3, and she discovered that by taking a tiny dose of medication, 7.5 mcg of this hormone every twelve hours, she sustained remarkable improvement. Within a few months, Ellie's energy level had improved to the point that she was ready to discontinue her thyroid medication completely. She reported that she was really pleased with her progress and felt that her energy had returned to normal.

Here is an excellent example of how a simple trial of a tiny dose of thyroid medication, even in the face of normal thyroid blood tests, produced impressive results that could not have been achieved unless we had given it a chance.

## IODINE DEFICIENCY: THE NEW FRONTIER

Symptoms of iodine deficiency include an enlarged thyroid (known as a goiter), hypothyroidism (with its attendant symptoms of fatigue, weakness, constipation, depression, dry skin, brittle hair and nails, cold sensitivity, abnormalities of the menstrual cycle, weight gain, and protruding eyes), fibrocystic breast disease, miscarriages, and stillbirths.

For those of you who live in the Midwest, it has long been known that iodine deficiency is rampant. The soil in this region is so severely depleted in iodine that crops grown on this soil and the animals that feed on those crops are all iodine deficient. Nearly 100 years ago, medical professionals realized that the common presence of an enlarged thyroid gland in the form of a goiter was due primarily to this deficiency of iodine. To counter it, iodine was added to salt, creating iodized salt. The incidence of goiters diminished greatly, and we reached a place where everyone just knew that iodized salt had to be a part of our daily lives.

This practice continued for decades, until the 1980s, when cardiologists began to emphasize the possible problems of consuming too much salt, most notably because of its effects on high blood pressure and heart disease. At about the same time, bread manufacturers removed iodine from their product (where it was used as a preservative) and replaced it with bromide. Over time, what we created for ourselves was a double whammy of a health dilemma. We now have a serious situation where iodine intake has once again dropped dramatically, especially in the Midwest. An informal poll of my patients, most of whom are holistically oriented, shows that more than 90 percent of them mostly consume sea salt. While perhaps a healthier form of salt, sea salt also does not contain iodine. The other part of this double whammy is that our environment now contains large amounts of fluoride and bromide. Both of these elements are so similar in structure to iodine that they bind to the sites in the body that require iodine and essentially block it from functioning. So we have evolved to a situation where we have inadequate amounts of iodine in our diet, and the small amount that we do take in cannot function properly because of the presence of fluoride and bromide.

Until recently, we have not had the ability to accurately test for iodine levels in our bodies. But over the past several years, a few labs have developed the *iodine load test,* which enables us to learn with a great deal of accuracy whether patients are deficient in this key element and to what extent. The test is relatively simple to perform: Patients take a measured oral dose of iodine with potassium iodide, and then collect all of their urine specimens for twenty-four hours. If they have a sufficient amount of iodine in their bodies already, then the dose we give them will pass right through their system and into their urine. If they are deficient, their bodies will grab the iodine it needs, and that iodine will not make it into the urine. A normal test would show that 90 percent or more of the iodine administered made it into the patient's urine. Anything less than 90 percent denotes varying degrees of deficiency. Another good test is collecting an overnight urine specimen and analyzing it for iodine content.

In my own practice, I have found that more than 90 percent of my patients are significantly iodine deficient. Replacing the iodine is simple and often produces great clinical improvement.

Iodine is taken up by the body mostly through the thyroid gland, so any thyroid imbalance should also address the patient's iodine needs. That is why I am including this discussion in this chapter. The other major tissue of the body that needs iodine is the breast. It is less commonly appreciated that breast problems may require iodine replacement as well. This is true for fibrocystic breast disease and for the prevention and treatment of breast cancer as well.

Recent research suggests that our body needs iodine in every cell for optimal metabolism. As our knowledge about iodine deficiency expands, I suspect we will be looking at a global problem, not unlike the one that existed 100 years ago. We will need to relearn how to add iodine back into our diet.

However, we do need to be careful with our use of iodine; too large a dose (especially in the presence of a damaged gland) may lead to additional irritation of the thyroid gland. Even in the face of deficiency, more is not always better, and once again I implore you to work with a knowledgeable professional to do this correctly.

## ESTELLE'S STORY

Estelle was forty-seven years old when she came to me because of her struggles with fibromyalgia and chronic fatigue. She had many of the problems that accompany fibromyalgia, including irritable bowel syndrome, depression, and menopausal symptoms. She had symptoms that suggested that mold toxicity might be part of this constellation as well.

Estelle's health did improve noticeably with the complete treatment approach utilized in our office. However, she was still not well enough to return to work, was barely functioning, and was somewhat depressed. When I performed the Iodine Load Test, I discovered that her levels of excretion were only 59 percent (normal is 90 percent or more). Within six weeks of starting iodine and potassium iodide (Iodoral), Estelle was markedly better. Her depression lifted, and her energy level improved to such an extent that she was able to resume full-time work.

I hope that you're beginning to see how the functional medicine model works: We analyze, step-by-step, the likeliest imbalances in the body, treat them, and see how the individual responds. With each positive response, we add another piece to our understanding of the imbalance puzzle. If the patient does not respond to our intervention, we stop treatment and go back to the drawing board to come up with the next viable puzzle piece. The vast majority of our patients are far too complicated for one single treatment to cure them. Instead, we keep building on our successful treatments until the patient has crested some threshold, unique to them, and becomes well. What I mean by "threshold" is that in chronically ill individuals, there are usually so many biochemical imbalances that fixing just one of them is not sufficient to provide healing. When we have addressed enough of those imbalances (anywhere from two to twenty) their bodies have finally gotten enough of their biochemical needs met that they can now push forward into wellness using their innate healing abilities. Unless this threshold is reached, we fall short of engaging those natural healing abilities.

## FURTHER READING

Arem, Ridha. *The Thyroid Solution: A Revolutionary Mind-Body Program for Regaining Your Emotional and Physical Health*. New York: Ballantine Books, 2007.

Brownstein, David. *Iodine: Why You Need It, Why You Can't Live Without It*. 2nd ed. West Bloomfield, MI: Medical Alternatives Press, 2006.

Wilson, E. Dennis. *Wilson's Thyroid Syndrome: A Reversible Thyroid Problem*. 4th ed. Rice, WA: Cornerstone Publishing, 1991.

## CHAPTER 6

# Sex Hormone Imbalances

## Now That I Have Your Attention . . .

I'm afraid this chapter won't be as racy as the title suggests. In fact, the way sex hormones work in your body is quite similar to how some of the other hormones we've already talked about, like the thyroid and adrenal hormones, work in your body. Simply put: You need them, and you need them in exactly the right amounts. This is not one of those cases where more is better. Thyroid balance is perhaps a more obvious example because we know that taking too much of that hormone is not good, but having too little isn't good for us either. Like Goldilocks's porridge, hormone levels have to be *just right*. Sex hormones follow this same model.

### ESTROGEN DEFICIENCY FOR WOMEN

Certain tissues in our bodies are designed to interact with hormones preferentially. That is, these tissues have specially constructed landing sites called *receptors*, each of which is designed to respond to specific hormones and not much else. For example, in women there are receptors for the estrogen hormones located in the brain, heart, and vaginal tissues. These receptive tissues *need* estrogen in order to function properly. Without it, the brain simply doesn't work as it should, and when estrogen levels are low, we see the symptoms of estrogen deficiency.

Several times a year I will see a woman who has seen her cardiologist for heart palpitations but has received no solutions to that problem. Often, when we provide estrogen for a measured deficiency in that hormone, the palpitations disappear. Likewise, vaginal dryness is frequently

---

### Symptoms of Estrogen Deficiency

- Hot flashes
- Night sweats
- Mood swings
- Depression
- Insomnia
- Vaginal dryness
- Urinary frequency and urgency
- Decreased libido (sex drive)
- Heart palpitations
- Fatigue
- Cognitive impairment (difficulties with focus, memory, and concentration)

---

the result of the body lacking enough estrogen to meet the needs of those tissues. And while hot flashes and night sweats get a lot of press and attention, even more important are focus, concentration, memory, sleep, energy, and mood issues. To put it a bit differently: Hot flashes are really annoying at times, and many women do suffer through them quite terribly, but a woman's inability to think properly or sleep well or her sudden, inexplicable outbursts at others are, medically speaking, far more serious problems. Just think of it: A woman who is irritable when she knows she has no reason to be, who cries over small things, who is depressed and can't sleep, and who cannot think clearly or truly function in her daily life, has a serious but readily treatable problem. In terms of health, being able to function normally is not a luxury, but a necessity—as any woman who is going through this will tell you.

We have, of course, been aware of menopausal difficulties for centuries. In ancient China, menopausal women would drink the urine of pregnant women to treat menopausal symptoms (pregnancy results in a dramatic increase in estrogen production, which is excreted in the urine). However, in our current medical climate, these hormones have become charged with a great deal of misinformation. Many women (and men) are reluctant to take hormones because some physicians have suggested that they will be at a higher risk for a host of serious diseases. The most current concern is that estrogen will cause cancer, especially of the breast, and bring patients closer to heart attacks, strokes, and gallbladder disease. Let's be clear about what is being discussed.

Several years ago it was finally accepted that Premarin, the most widely prescribed medication in the United States, was clearly associated with a significant increase in breast cancer and blood clots. I say "finally" because we had plenty of information about this link for many years prior. In fact, twelve years have passed since this alarming fact first came to light, and we've noted that the incidence of breast cancer has dropped by almost 20 percent! Premarin, short for PREgnant MARes' urINe, is actually a synthetic material, a third of which consists of several types of naturally occurring human estrogens, while the other two-thirds consist of mostly horse estrogens called *equilins*. So for years doctors had been giving huge numbers of women synthetic materials, most of which were foreign to their metabolism. They compounded that prescription by adding synthetic progesterone, also foreign to women's metabolism. Why should we be surprised that this concoction we recommended to women for years turned out to be an unhealthy combination of synthetic hormones?

News of the dangerous side effects of synthetic hormones finally came to light, and it scared millions of women. The medical profession made a complete reversal of position. For years previously, the profession had implied that all women who were going through or had completed menopause needed to take these synthetic materials. Doctors believed that not only would these materials make menopause easier for women to tolerate, but that they would also protect women against heart disease and perhaps Alzheimer's disease. As we know now, they do nothing of the sort. Hormones are an integral part of a very fragile, delicate balance in the body. So why would an unnatural, synthetic chemical be of such great benefit? When the medical profession suddenly stopped prescribing these materials, women got scared. Many, without even consulting their physicians, stopped their synthetic hormones cold. Medical professionals scrambled for an answer for those millions of women who were now struggling with the frightening symptoms listed earlier. The best immediate answer for many women, according to conventional medicine, was to take a particular type of antidepressant—specifically, what are called *selective serotonin reuptake inhibitors* or SSRIs for short. (Prozac is an example of a SSRI.) This was the pharmaceutical industry's answer for millions of women suffering from estrogen deficiency. While those medications can, indeed, help somewhat with the symptoms of depression, mood swings, sleep, and hot flashes and night sweats, they are purely symptomatic treatments; what a woman's body needs is estrogen, and these medications are but a weak substitute for the real thing. Conventional medicine has not entirely abandoned Premarin, but now knowing its risks, reserves it for use only in the most severely afflicted women.

There is another answer to this problem, and it is one that conventional medicine has been slow to embrace, again for reasons I cannot fathom. We have available, and have for many years, *natural hormones:* estrogens, progesterone, and testosterone, which are concocted and made available through compounding pharmacies. These materials are now commonly referred to as *bioidentical* hormones, meaning that they are biochemically identical to the hormones our bodies make for us. Bioidentical hormones are generally extracted from plants, which, surprisingly, produce the same hormones we do. These bioidentical hormones have not been studied as long and carefully as the synthetics; in fact, I don't anticipate that they will be, since research dollars come primarily from the pharmaceutical industry, and you cannot patent—thus make huge profits from—natural materials. The research we do have, however, indicates that the bioidentical materials are much safer and better tolerated than the synthetics. From my perspective, that makes a great deal of sense, as natural materials would obviously suit the body's needs more effectively than would synthetics.

I personally view hormone replacement as a physical need that must be met. All symptoms are just the body's way of telling its owner that something is not right and something must be done. How could that be wrong? I've provided natural hormone replacement for more than twenty years, and my experience is that it is very safe, very well tolerated, and very necessary. Why would anyone take an antidepressant when her body really needs estrogen? I cannot count the number of women I've treated who are living comfortable, productive, and healthy lives using natural hormones. This includes those who had done poorly on synthetic hormones, as well as those who have chosen to go directly to the bioidentical materials.

One unique aspect to my prescribing of natural hormones—which has never been characteristic of conventional approaches to synthetic hormones—is that I start by measuring the current hormone levels with a simple blood test. Most physicians have found that blood testing of these hormones is much more accurate than salivary testing. That, too, is my experience. This blood test gives me a precise idea of what the patient needs. I can then write a prescription for exactly that amount of hormone, and this prescription will be filled by a compounding pharmacy. This precision is really helpful. For many years, Premarin came in only two dosage strengths: 0.6 mg and 1.25 mg. This never made sense to me. Given the biochemical uniqueness of all women and of all people in general, how could only two choices of dosage meet all of their individual needs? Years later, Premarin was made available in two additional dosages of 0.3 mg and 0.9 mg. Even so, only four dosage strengths for all women?

After we measure the levels of the three estrogens—estriol (E3), estradiol (E2), and estrone (E1)—as well as progesterone and testosterone, we can design a natural hormone replacement that precisely puts that woman back into balance. Philosophically, it makes sense to me that meeting a woman's personal, unique hormonal needs is a healthy thing to do, and my experience reveals that this is true. Women who were unable to take Premarin for a variety of reasons, including migraine headaches, joint pain, and a host of more subtle side effects, can usually take the natural materials with no side effects at all.

We still have much to learn. How to formulate these bioidentical hormones is an area of debate among physicians. I've noticed that capsules work best for most of my patients. Some physicians prescribe the hormones as capsules designed to be placed into the cheek and left until they dissolve, which are called *troches*. Other physicians administer the hormones using topical creams, but many of us have found that absorption of hormone from the skin is quite variable, and I've found that topical creams are not as reliable or predictable as capsules. Nevertheless, natural hormones are much safer than synthetics and much more appreciated by a person who needs them to function, no matter the form in which they are taken.

As with any hormonal treatment protocol, the patient needs to be followed carefully by someone trained in using these materials. Individuals should never begin any natural hormonal treatment without the supervision of a knowledgeable clinician or medical practitioner. In this digital age, it is possible to go online and have bioidentical hormones shipped to you without putting a healthcare provider in the loop. I've had patients come to me already taking these materials, and they are usually struggling because they had no idea about dosage or balance. Again, this makes little sense to me. You wouldn't take thyroid hormones or insulin without an expert's guidance. Why should taking estrogen be any different?

## PROGESTERONE AND TESTOSTERONE FOR WOMEN

Having focused on estrogen thus far, let's expand our discussion into the other sex hormones, first with women, then with men.

All hormonal health is about *balance*. Somehow, the public has gotten the idea that it's all related to estrogen levels only. When a woman is in her prime, hormonal health involves every one of her hormones, so why would that change when she gets older? The time in which a body is moving into menopause but hasn't quite gotten there is called *perimenopause*. We have learned that this stage involves an imbalance called *estrogen dominance*. In fully evolved menopause, we see clear estrogen deficiency, but before the ovaries stop making much estrogen, there is a time in which it makes even less progesterone. When this occurs, symptoms arise because there is way too much estrogen *relative* to progesterone. The estrogen is dominant, the balance is tipped, and this is quite unhealthy. Many women who experience this assume that they just aren't making enough estrogen, but actually the reverse is true. When we evaluate this balance by hormone testing, we can provide natural progesterone until the hormonal balance shifts into true estrogen deficiency.

Again, for reasons that are unclear to me, we have long underestimated the importance of progesterone. For example, when a woman undergoes a hysterectomy and is clearly in need of hormone replacement, she is usually prescribed only estrogen. It was assumed for many years that progesterone's only real function was to assist in the sloughing of the uterine lining that built up during the luteal phase of the menstrual cycle. Without a uterus, why give progesterone? It turns out, however, that progesterone is an important precursor for other hormones, especially adrenal hormones; it helps to calm the nervous system; it stimulates new bone growth (important for those with osteoporosis); it improves libido; and it regulates the sensitivity of estrogen receptors. It is time to recognize the value of progesterone and include it in all of our discussions.

We can also measure testosterone, which is needed primarily for energy and sex drive. With our blood tests of hormonal levels, we can custom-make a prescription that will enable our patient to move into balance, and I believe that this translates into good health.

Many women fear that they will have to take hormones forever. This is rarely the case. Most find that after several years they have outgrown the need for hormones and will not need them again. Part of the process of treatment is for the patient to periodically stop taking hormones to see how she responds. Her body will tell her, quite clearly, whether or not she still needs the bioidentical hormone prescription.

It is also helpful for patients to be aware of the important interaction of estrogen with thyroid hormones, the adrenal hormones, and with serotonin and dopamine. This means that we shouldn't look at any one hormone in isolation, but only in relationship to other hormones. We must maintain balance. These are biochemical dominoes. One deficiency begins, affects another, and then another, and then another. These hormones are an important and integral part of our Big Six approach to the evaluation of biochemical imbalances in the body.

## KRISTY'S STORY

Kristy was forty-three years old when she came to see me several years ago, and she had a very simple request: "Fix me." She told me that she had been on low doses of thyroid hormone for twenty-two years, but she still felt like she had all the symptoms of thyroid deficiency. The most prominent of these was extreme fatigue. She described lying around in bed all day without much movement. On a bad day, she would get up and try to do laundry, pay bills, and clean her house. But this would end up exhausting her. "My body throbs and I have muscle pain all the time," she told me.

When Kristy awoke in the mornings, she said it felt as if she had been beaten with a baseball bat all night. It often took her until noon for her to be able to get up and get dressed. She did not have hot flashes or night sweats, but she did have significant problems with focus, memory, and concentration. She also had vaginal dryness and an unusually low sex drive. She admitted that she was irritable and angry all of the time and felt depressed.

The problem was that she knew she had nothing to be depressed about.

Kristy had undergone a hysterectomy eleven years earlier, but her ovaries had been left intact. It is quite frequent after any gynecological surgery for an early menopause to ensue, but most physicians believe that it's nearly impossible for a woman to begin her menopause until she is in her late forties. Unfortunately, these complaints of early menopause often go unrecognized and unheeded.

The standard test used by conventional medicine to determine the presence of menopause is called the follicle-stimulating hormone (FSH) test, but many physicians are unaware that this test may not yield positive results until five to eight years after menopause has actually begun! This huge chunk of time allows for the diagnosis to be missed, and the opportunity to help that unfortunate patient is lost in the confusion.

For Kristy, laboratory testing showed low progesterone, estriol, and DHEA levels. I supplemented her with 25 mg of DHEA each morning, and I also put her on a compounded prescription of estriol and progesterone to increase those levels. Her thyroid testing came back entirely normal. This was interesting, as she had been taking thyroid hormone for so long.

When she came back for her six-week follow-up visit, Kristy told me that she was doing really well, about 85 percent better than before. She had gone off the thyroid supplements without any negative effects, so it was clear that her rapid improvement was due to the use of female hormones and DHEA. She only got sore or tired after really overdoing it and essentially felt she was close to being cured in just six weeks.

---

## TESTOSTERONE IN MEN

There is also a male menopause, although it receives much less attention and is appropriately called andropause. Men also have estrogen and progesterone in their bodies, but in far smaller concentrations than women. For a variety of reasons, one of them being the excess aromatase enzyme made in fat cells (aromatase enzymes convert male sex hormones into estrogen), men may convert some of their testosterone into estrogen. When this happens, their hormone balance is altered. Too much estrogen can affect male sexual functioning, and just as importantly, energy and stamina. A little known but vital fact is that a great deal of research shows a man's testosterone level profoundly affects his heart. The higher the testosterone level, the less likely a man is to have a heart attack.

We continue to be deluged with advertisements for Viagra, Cialis, and Levitra. These medicines have, indeed, enabled many men to function sexually at a much higher level, and they are quite useful in that respect. But they don't help the body to make more testosterone, which is often what it really needs.

So, as with women, we need to be measuring testosterone levels in men, as well as estrogen levels and other binding proteins that allow us to determine what the true balance point is. Then, we can provide natural hormonal replacement when indicated. Unfortunately, many athletes have abused the use of testosterone and its precursors, so the FDA has made testosterone a *scheduled* drug, placing it in the same class of prescriptions as narcotics. In no way does that change the bio-

| Common Symptoms of Testosterone Deficiency | |
| --- | --- |
| Fatigue, tiredness | Mood swings |
| Decreased stamina | Hot flashes |
| Decreased libido (sex drive) | Palpitations |
| Erectile dysfunction | Insomnia |
| Muscle weakness | Inability to concentrate |
| Depression | Antisocial tendencies |

chemical need for testosterone that a man may require to achieve normal hormone levels.

In this culture, it is perfectly acceptable for women to discuss their hormone balance with their doctors. Unfortunately, there is a stigma around or reluctance about men doing the same. I suspect that many men would live much healthier lives if they could just understand that these are natural biochemical alterations, and that there is as little shame in noting sexual changes as there is in noting the onset of diabetes. Both need treatment. Alas, many men suffer not only sexual dysfunction, which they will not discuss with anyone—doctor or best friend—but they also experience the consequences of lower energy levels, decreased stamina, and muscle weakness, which are just as serious.

## SHELDON'S STORY

Sheldon came to see me at the age of forty-two. Initially, his symptoms consisted of extreme fatigue and an overall sense of feeling poorly. We quickly realized that he had developed adult-onset diabetes mellitus, and with conventional treatment he rapidly improved. But after several months, he was still aware of residual fatigue, poor stamina, and a decreased sex drive with moderate erectile dysfunction. When we tested his testosterone level, it was quite low at 178 ng/dL (normal level is 241–827 ng/dL). I have often found that in younger men, the indiscriminate use of testosterone as a prescription medication may, because of its biofeedback loops with the pituitary gland, actually shut down the production of testosterone and paradoxically make the problem worse. (A biofeedback loop is simply a mechanism in which the body believes it has enough of a hormone because the person is taking that hormone and so it sends itself a message to stop producing it.) Instead, I provided Sheldon with a prescription for a small dose of Clomid, 10 mg, taken three times weekly, which stimulates the testes to make more testosterone. Follow-up measurements of his testosterone levels showed that they had come back into the middle of the normal range, and he reported immediate improvement in energy, stamina, and sexual function. (His wife, also a patient of ours, thanked me too.)

As you can see, investigating sex hormone balances in *both* men and women is another central feature of our functional medicine program.

## FURTHER READING

Morgenthaler, John, and Jonathan V. Wright. *Natural Hormone Replacement for Women Over 45.* Petaluma, CA: Smart Publications, 1997.

Shippen, Eugene. *The Testosterone Syndrome: The Critical Factor for Energy, Health, and Sexuality—Reversing the Male Menopause.* New York: M. Evans and Company, 2001.

Vliet, Elizabeth. *Screaming to Be Heard: Hormonal Connections Women Suspect, and Doctors Still Ignore.* 2nd ed. New York: M. Evans and Company, 2000.

CHAPTER 7

# Food Allergies

---

## Nothing to Sneeze At

You might think it's somewhat obvious: The food we eat, the water we drink, and the air we breathe play an especially significant role in our overall health. Unfortunately, the basic concepts of nutrition and digestion, as well as their importance to health, are not only given little attention in medical school education, but they are often neglected or ignored in current clinical practice. When people ask their doctors about these subjects, they are frequently given the impression that their diet doesn't matter much. But it does matter—a lot. These patients realize that their doctors don't always have the information that they are seeking. But why not? Aren't they medical specialists?

Over the next few chapters, I would like to discuss several medical concepts that are not parts of conventional medicine. These include food allergies; the overgrowth of toxic microorganisms (bacteria, yeast, and parasites) in the intestinal tract; and how food may stimulate the overproduction of insulin in the form of hypoglycemia (low blood sugar). First, we turn to food allergy.

## FOOD ALLERGIES: IMMEDIATE FOOD SENSITIVITY VS. DELAYED SENSITIVITY

There are several different kinds of food allergy. Each is unique because of the various antibodies produced by the body in response to its reaction to a particular food. All of our allergies crop up based on how our immune system reacts to a specific material, usually a protein. There are five specific and different kinds of antibodies that the body can create, and they are all called *immunoglobulins*. They are differentiated by letters, so we call them immunoglobulin A (IgA), as well as IgD, IgE, IgG, and IgM.

Perhaps the most common type of food reaction with which most of us are familiar occurs when someone consumes a particular product (commonly seafood, strawberries, or peanuts) and then breaks out in hives within fifteen to twenty minutes. This alarming reaction by the immune system is brought about by the specific immunoglobulin IgE. All physicians acknowledge the importance and existence of this reaction. If severe, in fact, this reaction can result in life-threatening conditions in which the lips and tongue swell up and the ability to breathe becomes compromised. We call these types of responses *immediate sensitivity reactions*. They constitute medical emergencies and must be treated as such.

More common in patients, but much less known within our profession, are the *delayed sensitivity reactions*, which are mediated primarily by immunoglobulins IgM and IgG. These reactions can produce a wide array of symptoms and illness with the delay ranging from six hours to three days. (See Common Symptoms of Delayed Sensitivity to Food below.) This delay makes these reactions much harder to diagnose because most of us don't remember what we ate three days ago and are not likely to attribute what we're feeling today to something that we consumed that long ago. These reactions, however, are quite prevalent.

## Common Symptoms of Delayed Sensitivity to Food

| | |
|---|---|
| Fatigue | Eczema |
| Cognitive difficulties | Psoriasis |
| Arthritis or arthraligia (joint pain) | Cholecystitis |
| Myalgia (muscle pain) | Urinary frequency and pain |
| Bronchospasms | Heart palpitations |
| Inflammatory bowel disease | Autoimmune disease |
| Allergic rhinitis | Enuresis (bed-wetting) |
| Irritable bowel syndrome (IBS) | Sinusitis |

## CLARENCE'S STORY

Clarence was a seventy-four-year-old gentleman who came to me several years ago complaining of a sudden increase in joint pain, which was diagnosed by his family physician as arthritis. Along with his joint pain, which he experienced all over his body, he also noted an increase in fatigue and poor concentration. I asked Clarence if he was eating more of any particular foods than usual. He responded that since it was summer and fresh corn and tomatoes were now available in abundance from his garden, he was eating those foods almost every night. As these are common allergic foods, I suggested that he stop eating tomatoes and corn for ten days. It usually takes three days for the intestinal tract to clear what is already in it from recent meals, so I cautioned him that he might not see any results for that time. I indicated to him that if these foods were indeed the cause of his symptoms, he should experience rapid improvement by eliminating their intake. At his next visit he informed me that, to his surprise, his symptoms had resolved completely.

I then instructed Clarence to test these foods separately by eating a lot of one of the two food we suspected as his allergic culprit with every meal for three days. If he did not react, he could try the next food. If he did react, he should wait for three days to clean his system out and then try the next food. He discovered that he reacted to both of them. Tomatoes and corn brought his symptoms back with full force, but those symptoms disappeared again when he stopped eating those foods. Not only did his joint pain vanish, but he had much more energy, and his concentration came back to normal as well. This is an excellent example of classical delayed food allergy.

## Food Allergies: Diagnosis and Treatment

I would estimate that at least 50 percent of all joint and muscle pain is caused by food allergies, and when the offending foods are discovered and their consumption discontinued, many people feel much, much better. This means that a great deal of what is commonly diagnosed as osteoarthritis or degenerative arthritis is actually caused by a food sensitivity. It also means that it is readily treated by discovering the offending foods and avoiding them. The diagnosis of *arthritis* is far overused by physicians, which is quite unfortunate. It is defined to patients as an inflammation of the joint, with the implication that it is permanent and ultimately destructive to that joint. *Arthritis* is a frightening word that creates pictures of lifelong suffering in patients' minds. As I am implying here, however, this is actually not always the case, since joint pain caused by a reaction to food goes away readily and completely when the offending substance is removed from the diet. A more precise medical term for this form of joint pain would be *arthralgia*, which simply means "joint pain," and does not carry the implications of destructive, eternal, or long-lasting pain. Occasionally, medical practitioners unwittingly cause additional suffering to their patients with an imprecise use of language, and this is a good example of how that can happen.

The most common foods incriminated in delayed food allergy reactions are cow's milk and wheat, followed in terms of frequency of reactions by sugar, corn in all of its various forms, and citrus products. Additional foods that can often specifically affect joint pain are pork and the nightshade family of plants, which includes tomatoes, potatoes, eggplant, and green peppers. Although Clarence's story involved the symptom of joint pain for these delayed allergies, please keep in mind that any, or even several, of the symptoms listed in Common Symptoms of Delayed Sensitivity to Food (see page 75) could result from delayed food allergies and can be responsive to evaluation and treatment.

Once delayed food allergy is suspected or considered as a possible component of any illness, there are several ways to make a clear and accurate diagnosis. The simplest and least expensive method, though not necessarily the easiest, is to embark on what we call an elimination diet, which I explained in Clarence's story earlier. This type of diet consists of eliminating all of the most likely offending foods and observing what happens over time. Typically we continue this elimination process for seven to ten days. As I also said earlier, the first three days of this diet are unlikely to give us much information, since the intestines have not yet expelled all of what is already in the system. So we really focus on the four to seven days after the elimination diet has begun. All I ask my patients to do is observe how they feel on this diet. If their symptoms improve or resolve significantly, this means that one or more of the foods we've eliminated is causing those symptoms, and we have established food allergy as a probable diagnosis for their illness. From here on, we have to play Sherlock Holmes to figure out which food or foods are the culprits.

Usually we eliminate all of the likeliest offenders at once. This means that I ask patients to stop consuming all milk products, wheat and corn in all forms, sugar, citrus, and any other food they suspect may be contributing to their symptoms. When I present this plan to my patients, some say that they would rather do one food at a time to make the process a bit easier for them. But I discourage this. The reason for encouraging individuals to discontinue all of the likeliest foods at the same time is that many patients have *multiple* food allergies. For example, if a person is allergic to both milk and wheat, and she eliminated the wheat but continued to consume milk, she could miss the benefits of being off wheat because the milk was still producing an overriding allergic reaction. Although it is a bit more troublesome for the patient to simultaneously eliminate all possible offending foods, it is a much more accurate method for evaluating their response.

If after seven to ten days, with a careful and meticulous elimination diet, the patient notes no improvement whatsoever, it is unlikely that those foods are a part of the problem, and I then encourage the patient to resume his usual diet. This does not completely rule out food allergy as a part of the problem, but it does tell us about those specific foods we just tested.

On the other hand, if the patient is clearly better (not necessarily cured, as there may be other components to the symptoms), then we must determine what foods are responsible. The simple rule I work with is for the patient to add back one new food, lots of it, in pure form, every three days. Let's go over this in more detail. To ensure the highest level of accuracy, we test with only one food in pure form. By "pure form" I mean that if you are testing milk products, you can consume lots of milk, cream, yogurt, sour cream, or cottage cheese. But pure form milk products does not include foods such as ice cream, which contains sugar and flavorings. Eating nonpure foods would compromise the interpretation of the patient's response. Delayed food reactions, as I have noted, may take up to three days to show up, so we have to wait at least that long to be sure that no reaction has occurred. If a reaction occurs sooner, of course, the patient should discontinue that food immediately and wait three days to clear it out of his or her system before testing another food.

Delayed sensitivity reactions also require that *enough* of the tested food be eaten to produce a reaction, if there is going to be one. Tiny amounts may not produce a noticeable reaction. Along with the three-day delay, this is another reason that intelligent, thoughtful patients have not suspected food allergy as a component of their symptoms. For example, if patients eat Wheaties for breakfast, a sandwich for lunch, and pizza for dinner, they might not recognize that they are consuming a substantial amount of wheat. Smaller amounts of wheat, say just the sandwich for lunch, might not produce this reaction, which would throw otherwise observant patients offtrack. They might notice that sometimes they reacted to wheat and sometimes not. Quantity matters, especially when doing this type of testing.

Sometimes, less commonly consumed foods, even in trace amounts, are the culprits, and these can be difficult to diagnose. In the past, tests for food allergy, such as skin testing and radioallergosorbent (RAST) blood tests, have been used with varying degrees of accuracy. For example, since the majority of food allergy reactions are *delayed,* skin testing may not provide an accurate diagnosis if it is not followed by a full three days of observation (which is rarely done by most practitioners who perform skin testing). In recent years, ELISA technology has improved the situation considerably. (ELISA is short for enzyme-linked immunosorbent assay and ACT stands for Advanced Cell Technique.) The most accurate test I've found is the ELISA/ACT blood test performed by Dr. Russ Jaffe's laboratory. He uses a somewhat unique testing procedure on blood, evaluating for exposure to 380 common foods and 100 common household chemicals. By using the results produced by his laboratory, I've enabled many of my patients to improve or heal. Additionally, materials that are more difficult to test for, such as food coloring and additives, can be discovered with this test. For example, the chemical monosodium glutamate (MSG), frequently used as a meat tenderizer or flavor enhancer in Chinese restaurants and steakhouses, is a common allergen. Increasingly we find that Nutrasweet (aspartame) also causes delayed sensitivity reactions, especially in migraine sufferers. Dr. Jaffe published a paper on the prevalence of food allergy in fibromyalgia, noting that 73 percent of fibromyalgia patients had significant food allergies, and that their symptoms responded well to the elimination of the offending foods.

Dr. Alan McDaniel began his medical career as an ENT (ear, nose, and throat) surgeon, but discovered that by evaluating his patients for allergies, he was able to avoid surgery in most of them and has subsequently focused his practice on diagnosing and treating allergic conditions. (He later realized that these patients did even better when he also evaluated and treated their thyroid, adrenal, and sex hormone imbalances as well.) Dr. McDaniel has noted that skin testing can be quite helpful in making these diagnoses (and in providing a basis for treatment) if the testing is allowed to be evaluated three days after the skin tests are applied; unfortunately, this is rarely done.

## OLIVIA'S STORY

Olivia was seventy-six years old when she came to me with a twenty-five-year history of the inflammatory bowel disorder Crohn's disease. This condition can be a serious, life-threatening medical problem. She had been followed by gastroenterologists at the University of Kansas medical school, and she received all of the customary biopsies, clearly confirming the diagnosis, and underwent the customary treatments. Nevertheless, she had never done well with these conventional treatments. Upon testing her stool, I found pathogenic bacteria and yeast (infective microbes), which we treated (see Chapter 8). I also identified her food allergies and we removed those offending materials from her diet. Olivia's symptoms resolved completely for the first time in twenty-five years. She was absolutely thrilled. When she returned to her gastroenterologist for a follow-up colonoscopy, he found no trace of her bowel disease.

When Olivia described our treatment program to her gastroenterologist, who had followed her for years, he told her it was impossible that this treatment could have led to her remission. I guess it was possible that our treatment wasn't a factor in her healing. However, since she has continued to do extremely well, with no recurrence over the past eight years, I can be reasonably comfortable in concluding that her exceptional improvement occurred because we removed the allergic foods from her diet that were directly responsible for bringing on these symptoms. She still finds that if she mistakenly eats one of the foods she is sensitive to, she will have a short episode of symptoms; but no full-blown recurrence of inflammatory bowel disease has appeared.

## NORMA'S STORY

Norma first came to see me at the age of forty-two with the diagnosis of rheumatoid arthritis. She had been seeing a rheumatologist and three other physicians for the past several years, but over the past year had not responded to any of the eight or nine medications prescribed. She hurt all the time and she was frustrated. Norma was one of those unfortunate patients I see occasionally who had severe reflux problems from a sensitive stomach, and almost all the medications that had been used to treat her rheumatoid arthritis had caused those gastrointestinal symptoms to flare up intensely. She had gamely tried every medication available for treatment, but each one had severe, intolerable side effects. She was hoping that a completely different approach might be of value.

To digress for a moment from the subject of food allergy: We have found with rheumatoid arthritis, as with several other autoimmune conditions, that a number of alternative approaches are often helpful. As we describe here, looking for and treating food allergies is often an effective strategy. Additionally, looking for and treating heavy-metal toxicity is often of value, and the use of long-term, low dose minocin (an antibiotic in the tetracycline family) has been effective for some. Newer information about the benefits for the immune system by treating vitamin D deficiency has also emerged. And, as unusual as it sounds, there is a long history for using bee venom to treat this condition. There is even a report in the medical literature that describes the use of journaling as a treatment for the stress associated with autoimmune diseases. (See Chapter 21.) Patients spend twenty minutes a day, for just three days, writing down on paper a detailed account of their stressors and their feelings about those stressors. This simple procedure results in significant improvement for many patients, and fortunately for Norma she responded well to journaling. (See also Chapter 21 on autoimmunity.)

Another area of benefit to Norma was revealed when we cultured her stool (a diagnostic method that we will discuss at length in Chapter 8) and discovered the presence of the pathogenic bacteria Klebsiella and treated her for it. Klebsiella is especially associated with joint pain, so looking for and addressing it is often helpful for patients with that affliction. Not only can Klebsiella contribute to joint pain by producing infection, it can also produce joint pain from the release of toxins when it is killed by the body. Furthermore, a few patients are also allergic to this bacteria, and strategies that strengthen the immune system's ability to resist this allergic reaction may be curative for rheumatoid arthritis. (For more information, see Chapter 21 and the discussion of LDA [low-dose allergen] therapy.)

After completing and treating Norma's pathogen problem, we then utilized Dr. Jaffe's ELISA/ACT test, which showed that she had strong delayed reactions to aluminum, chocolate, cocoa, black tea, cinnamon, coconut, polysorbate 80 (a common food additive), tapioca, chili, orange, caraway seeds, saccharine, paprika, shrimp, cola, sage, basil, and several household chemicals. Let me point out here that not only can aluminum be a toxin, but here it was an allergen as well.

When she meticulously avoided all of the foods and chemicals denoted by her testing, Norma reported astounding improvement in her symptoms. For several years afterward, her rheumatoid arthritis was well controlled with careful monitoring of her diet and occasional treatments of osteopathic manipulation. When she would get a flare-up of symptoms, she often recognized that it was because of particular stressors. By utilizing the journaling technique for several days to let out these particular stressors, she would often feel much better.

---

As Dr. Jaffe has discovered, and I can confirm, many autoimmune diseases have a food-allergy component. Patients with rheumatoid arthritis, lupus, and multiple sclerosis have improved significantly—and some have even been cured—by uncovering this allergy component of their illness. In my experience, food allergy is one of the most commonly overlooked causes for a wide variety of symptoms. Countless children with eczema and asthma and enuresis (bed-wetting), and adults with joint pain and fatigue, headaches, colitis, and irritable bowel syndrome have greatly improved with this simple evaluation for food allergy. We will also look at the role food allergy plays in autism spectrum disorder in Chapter 22.

After the discussion and stories presented here, you can immediately begin to see how important food allergy's role is in causing or contributing to many chronic medical conditions. Many patients are astonished to learn that some of the foods that they regularly eat are actually a part of their problem, and that the simple expedient of avoiding these foods provides great benefit. We regularly observe, to our patients' frustration, that the most likely allergic foods are the ones that they identify as their favorites. Of all the health imbalances presented in this book, food allergy is one of the most common and is often easiest to address. It's truly a shame that its importance is not yet universally recognized.

## FURTHER READING

Breneman, James C. *Basics of Food Allergy.* 2nd ed. Springfield, IL: Charles C .Thomas Pub Ltd., 1984.

Crook, William G. *Tracking Down Hidden Food Allergies.* 2nd ed. Jackson, TN: McGraw-Hill Professional Publishing, 1980.

Jaffe, Russell A, and Deuster, Patricia A, A Novel Treatment for Fibromyalgia Improves Clinical Outcomes in a Community-Based Study, *Journal of Musculoskeletal Pain,* Vol. 6, pp. 133–149 (1998).

## CHAPTER 8

# Intestinal Dysbiosis: Imbalances of the Gastrointestinal System

---

## Alimentary, My Dear Watson

Another prevalent health imbalance that is generally overlooked by conventional medicine is that of *intestinal dysbiosis*. The word *dysbiosis* is from the Latin *dys*, for imbalance or abnormality and *biosis* for life-forms or microbes—in this case, those that normally inhabit our intestines. Hence, this difficult but accurate phrase—*intestinal dysbiosis*—means that the flora and fauna of our gut is out of balance. Essentially, I am referring to the complicated ecosystem of our gastrointestinal (GI) tract. Understanding the workings of this complex ecosystem helps us evaluate its imbalances so that we can improve or heal them.

### THE GASTROINTESTINAL TRACT

Although we don't usually think of it this way, our gut is really a giant open tube connected to the outside world through its front end (our mouth) and its back end (our rectum). We usually think of our intestines as being "inside" us, but since it is open-ended on both sides, you could also see it, from another perspective as outside of us. It cannot possibly be sterile or free from germs like the rest of our body because it is constantly in direct contact with the external environment. When we eat food or drink liquids, those materials mix with the secretions of this giant tube, allowing our body to digest and assimilate what it needs. Because our gut is not sterile—meaning that it is filled with bacteria and other germs—we have evolved a very complicated ecosystem that actually helps us in many ways as we interact with both good and bad bacteria, yeast, and other microorganisms that gain entry into this system.

Our body actually *needs* a significant quantity of good bacteria to populate the gastrointestinal tract for a variety of reasons. One, since the GI tract is a true ecosystem, the more numerous the beneficial bacteria there are in it, the less of a foothold there is for more toxic (*pathogenic*) bacteria to gain space or nutrients in which to grow. A second reason we need these good bacteria is because they manufacture a number of nutrients that we need to survive, such as vitamin B12. Rather than be concerned about the presence of these bacteria, we should instead know that they are an integral part of our healthy bodies—we coexist with them in a way that is beneficial to both of us: We need them, and they need us. If this system is disturbed or damaged, most commonly by our taking antibiotics that kill off large numbers of helpful bacteria, the ecosystem becomes imbalanced. Destroying these beneficial bacteria allows room for the pathogenic bacteria, yeasts, and parasites, to gain a toehold and grow. Depending on which species of pathogens infect us, we may experience a variety of gastrointestinal symptoms: heartburn, reflux, gas, bloating, distention, cramps, pain, diarrhea, or constipation. Additionally, many of these pathogens release toxins into our body that can cause us to feel systemically, or globally, ill. Fatigue, depression, joint pain, cognitive impairment, yeast infections, and headache are just of few of the symptoms that may be due to the out-of-balance growth of bacteria or yeast within our intestines.

Furthermore, approximately 60 percent of our immune system is connected to our gastrointestinal system. This portion of the immune

### Symptoms of Intestinal Dysbiosis

- Diarrhea
- Constipation
- Gas and bloating
- Heartburn and reflux
- Irritable bowel syndrome
- Joint pain
- Fatigue
- Recurrent yeast infections
- Depression
- Abdominal pain and/or cramping
- Cognitive impairment (difficulty with focus, memory, and concentration)

system is called the *gut-associated lymphoid tissue* (GALT). Surrounding our gut are large patches of lymphocytes (important immune cell lines) called *Peyer's patches,* which process any potentially harmful microbes. The Peyer's patches produce antibodies to invaders to create a major line of defense. When you think about it, it isn't surprising that our body places so much emphasis on an immune system so close to our gut. Remember, we are dealing with an open-ended tube to the outside world, a system that is constantly exposed to possibly infectious agents. It makes sense that our bodies would have evolved this elaborate arrangement for dealing with these potential dangers. Our body has surrounded its intestinal system with a good portion of its immune system, assigning to that system the specific mission of monitoring the gastrointestinal tract and defending it from the invasion of potentially harmful germs.

If the invading microorganisms produce toxins or create an infectious or inflammatory response in the intestinal cells, they can weaken the tight connections between the intestinal cells, which are an important form of protective barrier. Once these cell-to-cell connections have been loosened or opened by inflammation, the toxins can enter our body to do damage. This is also the mechanism by which food allergy occurs: We can only develop a food allergy if a foreign protein makes its way into our body without our blessing. The only way for these proteins to get across the barrier is to seep through the weakened cellular connections, which are supposed to be tight junctions. Other parts of our immune system are then forced to make antibodies to these proteins, hence causing food allergy. This disturbance in the tight junctions is often called *leaky gut.*

## THE SECOND BRAIN: OUR GUT

Another important and often underappreciated component of our gut physiology is called by some scientists our *second brain.* For many years, we have known that there is a larger concentration of neurotransmitters in the gut than there is in the brain. Neurotransmitters are chemicals that allow electrical impulses to be conducted from nerve cell to nerve cell, and we will discuss them at length in the section on amino acids in Chapter 13. Neurotransmitters include some chemicals about which you may have heard: serotonin, dopamine, and epinephrine. Recent research points to our intestinal tract as contributing to our mental well-being by producing these neurotransmitters, yet we still don't know exactly how this works. Old phrases such as "gut feeling" and "gut instinct" take on completely new meanings in this context.

These interactions in our intestinal system between good bacteria, the GALT, and neurotransmitters, create a complicated, interwoven system that we are just beginning to understand. The phrase *intestinal dysbiosis* is intended to convey some sense of that complexity and provides us with a great tool to analyze and understand it. Ultimately, this understanding can help us to heal, especially if this area has been neglected or damaged.

## THE INTESTINAL TRACT AS AN ECOSYSTEM

When I describe the gastrointestinal tract as an ecosystem, many of my patients look puzzled and confused. So allow me to use a bit of poetic license and paint a picture of what this ecosystem might look like. Imagine that your intestinal tract, both the small and large intestines, consists of miles and miles of white sandy beaches, with the ocean lapping up gently along its length. Populating these glorious beaches are thousands and thousands of happy families—the children diligently building sand castles while their parents wade into the surf or lay out on brightly colored beach towels. Imagine also the fringes of these beaches, way back in the dunes or hidden in small groves of trees behind the beach, where we might discover a few wild animals lying in wait—coyotes, raccoons, even a bear or two. These animals are extremely suspicious of the many humans roaming around, and they choose to remain in hiding. But when the sun finally sinks below the horizon, when the beaches are less populated, these beasts come out in search of food. In this picture, the people represent the good bacteria, consisting of many species of *Lactobacilli* and *Bifidobacteria,* the main species of good bacteria that populate our small intestine and large intestine, respectively. The wild animals represent different kinds of toxic species, such as *Candida* and pathogenic, or toxic, bacteria. This overall picture represents our healthy, normal state.

Now, imagine that something occurs to interfere with that perfect day at the beach—say a shark attacking a man while he surfs. Our happy families will leave the beach in droves, fearful that the shark might take another bite out of someone else. This mass exodus of people gives those wild animals complete and comfortable access to our beach. The indiscriminate use of antibiotics can be quite a shark attack for our body's beaches because they kill off so many good bacteria. What antibiotics leave behind are those wild animals, those creatures with no place else to go. In turn, the animals will eventually begin to grow and thrive. Our beaches will become populated by coyotes and raccoons and bears, and the families with their children will be very reluctant to come down to the beach ever again. The animals, those toxic species, have gained the upper hand.

When we attempt to rectify this situation, we use specific medications and herbs that could be seen as clearing the beach of all sharks. These treatments invite thousands of new families (a symbol for the use of probiotics) to come down to the beach and play. The wild animals have been happy at this beach for some time now, but they are now being driven off, slowly but surely. They migrate farther and farther down the beach until the families feel safe enough to return. That this is a slow and gradual process of change during treatment is important to understand: We can't simply get into beach jalopies and ride wildly onto the sands, shooting indiscriminately at the wildlife. Instead, we have to work *with* the system to restore it. As you might imagine, this does take some time. I hope this little analogy, although a bit fanciful, will help you to understand the concept of intestinal ecology.

## Diagnosing Intestinal Imbalances

In practice, when I encounter situations of intestinal imbalance, I first ask my patient to collect a stool specimen (a bit disgusting, but truly helpful), and I send it to a laboratory for analysis. Over the years, I've had excellent results from the Genova Diagnostics lab (formerly the Great Smokies Diagnostic Lab), but many others can provide these analyses as well. From the information derived from the stool specimen, I can determine whether or not the patient's body can make enough digestive enzymes and hydrochloric acid, or whether some form of malabsorption of certain food nutrients is taking place. Most importantly, from this analysis I can determine if there are normal amounts of good bacteria in the intestines, including *Lactobacilli,* the main beneficial bacteria of the small intestine (which many people associate with acidophilus), and *Bifidobacteria,* the main beneficial bacteria of the large intestines. From these test results, I can also evaluate for the presence of toxic or pathogenic bacteria, yeasts, and parasites. In a healthy person there should be plenty of both the *Lactobacilli* and *Bifidobacteria* (designated as 4+ on the lab report). If the individual has received significant exposure to antibiotics, even in the distant past, the antibiotic may have upset the delicate balance of the gut by killing off the good bacteria and leaving small amounts of toxic microbes behind to multiply. The overgrowth of this toxic bacteria or yeast can persist for years.

The toxic bacteria irritate, infect, or inflame the intestines, causing or contributing to irritable bowel disease, spastic colon, and inflammatory bowel diseases such as Crohn's disease and ulcerative colitis. Additionally, these microbes can release toxins into the patient's body that can contribute to chronic fatigue, brain fog, joint pain, and headaches. All of these symptoms are usually accompanied by an overriding sense of not feeling well, which goes well beyond simple bowel symptomatology. The good news is that the laboratory not only tells us which microbes are involved, but it also tests these microbes against the known antibiotics and natural remedies that could destroy them. This is similar to the well-known process that doctors use when patients report that they have a bladder infection. A sample of their urine is taken and tested for what are called "culture and sensitivities." That just means that doctors take the urine sample, place it on a culture plate, and set discs of the most useful antibiotics on top of the sample. The discs that clearly kill the growing bacteria obviously represent the antibiotics we want to use to treat that infection. In exactly the same manner, we can use culture techniques to determine the best treatments available for the specific microbe we find on our patient's stool test.

One of the things we've learned over the past several years is that these organisms that infect our bowel are mutating and becoming less and less sensitive to the medications we have used against them for a long time. In conventional medicine, the concept of *chronic yeast infection* is not considered a valid diagnosis when it refers to a species of *Candida* found in our intestinal tract (it can also occur in the vaginal area). As with other concepts discussed in this book—hypoglycemia, dental amalgam toxicity, chronic Lyme disease, chronic Epstein-Barr infection, and food allergy—the medical profession has somehow decided to ignore the presence of yeast in the gastrointestinal tract. Some do so by claiming that "everyone has small amounts of yeast," so it's nothing we need to pay attention to. Some have disparaged this concept by confusing it with *systemic yeast infection.* Systemic infections are caused by those yeasts that have gotten into the bloodstream and are delivering toxic microbes to every part of our body. Systemic yeast infections certainly exist, but they are very rare, and when present, they are life threatening. A patient with this type of infection requires intravenous antibiotics and hospitalization.

But this is not what we are discussing here; instead, we are discussing overgrowth of yeast and toxic bacteria—in the bowel specifically. While these overgrowths are not life threatening, the direct inflammatory effects of these microorganisms coupled with the release of toxins, which make their way through the bowel wall into the rest of our circulation, can make us feel pretty wretched. If these are not diagnosed and treated properly, we can feel this way for a very long time. Those physicians who maintain that these overgrowths are of no importance are missing an opportunity to make a big difference in their patients' intestinal health. To make this just a little more complicated, it is also possible to become *allergic* to some of these infecting organisms, such as *Candida* or *Klebsiella,* which we discussed in the previous chapter, and this adds yet another dimension to the pathological process, which needs to be a consideration in treatment.

Many patients associate the word *yeast* with vaginal yeast infections. While these infections are quite common, they are not exactly the same as intestinal yeast infections. Both cause patients to feel poorly; in one, the intestinal symptoms predominate, and in the other, vaginal symptoms predominate. The difference is that the "leaky gut" associated with dysbiosis allows toxins to be absorbed into the body and adds another level of toxicity for our patients. This does not happen with vaginal yeast infections.

Once again, it is by observing how patients respond to treatment that we can learn of the importance of this condition. Healing is not about theory; it's about results. I have personally treated several thousand patients who had an overgrowth of yeast from the intestinal system, and all of these cases were confirmed with the stool analysis. Nearly all of these patients report significant improvements in their symptoms when treated. If intestinal yeast is such a normal state of affairs, as many conventional doctors tend to believe, how could this healing be possible? When we repeat the stool tests of successfully treated patients, the *Candida* is no longer found. Might it still be present in minuscule amounts? Yes, it could be—and probably is. After years of looking at these results, I am strongly persuaded that any overgrowth noted on this test represents a nonphysiological state, and patients who demonstrate these laboratory results will benefit from treatment.

## Treating Intestinal Imbalances

The results of recent stool testing in our offices show that the yeasts are getting less responsive now to older treatments. As the media has been actively informing us, many species of bacteria are evolving in ways that make them nonresponsive to our usual antibiotics. Yeasts are doing the same thing. Years ago, a variety of simple supplements and herbs, such as capryllic acid, garlic, and berberine, were quite effective at killing intestinal yeast. But as we continue to observe the results of sensitivity tests, we find that some medications and herbs now rarely control these infections. Diflucan in particular, is increasingly less effective than it used to be, and we have to turn to stronger antifungal medications for results. Diflucan, which has been our old standby, no longer works in 10 to 15 percent of patients. Other stronger medications like Sporanox and Ketoconazole have become a necessity for successful treatment. Dr. Orian Truss, who pioneered the understanding and treatment of intestinal yeast conditions, believes that yeast rarely becomes tolerant to Nystatin and it is the cornerstone of his treatment program outlined in his classical book *The Missing Diagnosis*.

The key point I wish to make here is that by doing a simple stool test, which is covered by most health insurance companies, we can identify and treat these infections with precision. We simply follow the sensitivities provided by the laboratory and then add back the nutrients and supplements that we identify as deficient. Usually treatment involves adding probiotics, enzymes, or hydrochloric acid, accompanied by a change in the patient's diet.

## PROBIOTICS

*Probiotics* are various combinations of good bacteria, like the *Lactobacilli* and *Bifidobacteria* mentioned above. There are hundreds of species of these bacteria. We are becoming increasingly aware of how important this balance of good bacteria is to our health. Ideally, a probiotic preparation would match the exact balance of good bacteria that we were born with (which is unique to each of us). Unfortunately, since none of us had that tested at birth, the best probiotic choices would be those with the widest variety of bacterial species, so that our bodies could pick and choose those that matched our individual needs the best.

Many probiotics (and be aware that commercial probiotics may exist in a bewildering array of different species) may also include additional ingredients to improve the body's ability to nurture these good bacteria; these extra ingredients are sometimes referred to as *prebiotics.* These include fructooligosaccharides (FOS) and the benign yeast *Saccharomyces boulardii.*

When it comes to treating intestinal imbalances with probiotics and prebiotics especially, a trained, knowledgeable health professional is needed. Some of the pathogenic bacteria we are trying to defeat (such as *Klebsiella*) thrive on FOS, for example, and the incorrect or indiscriminate use of certain probiotics and prebiotics without testing can lead to serious problems. It should not come as a surprise that doctors can treat the condition with more precision if they know exactly which bacteria and yeast are involved. When it comes to balanced health, the bottom line keeps coming down to this: A clear and concise diagnosis is necessary for an appropriate treatment. Otherwise we are just shooting in the dark, and we might get lucky or we might not. Why shoot in the dark when light is available?

As noted, there are a bewildering number of probiotic formulations and an equal number of opinions on how to make the best use of them. Many beneficial bacterial species present in probiotics are killed, or mostly killed, by stomach acid. This means that a large proportion of these bacteria, if ingested in tablet or powder form, do not reach their intended destination alive. It also means that when my patients tell me that they are getting plenty of good bacteria in the commercial yogurt and acidophilus milk they consume, they may be mistaken. When we look at their stool tests, many are surprised to discover how few good bacteria are actually present when they have made extensive use of these products. Logic and experience suggest that the best way to deliver these beneficial bacteria to our intestines would be through an enteric-coated capsule. This protective covering ensures that the capsule goes through the stomach acid unscathed and dissolves in the intestines, placing the beneficial bacteria exactly where they need to be.

A common form of delivery of these bacteria is through freeze-dried bacteria. These bacteria are processed so that they are not really alive until they are reconstituted in the intestines. While many of the makers of these products claim superb reconstitution, our stool tests do not bear this out.

The best results seem to come from the use of *live culture* bacteria, which, by definition, require refrigeration. These are not as convenient as the freeze-dried form, which can sit out at room temperature for long periods of time, but in my opinion the freeze-dried variety are nowhere near as effective as the live bacteria. As noted above, products with the widest array of bacterial species tend to be the most effective.

We each have unique biochemistries, so it is important that we use our bodies as laboratories—in a sense—in which we discover what foods and what kind of diet are best for us. At some point you may wish to explore such diverse diets as the carbohydrate-specific diet, the low-oxalate diet, the Weston-Price diet, the Paleolithic diet, the GAPS diet, or macrobiotics, looking for what makes you the most comfortable. Keep in mind that your needs may change over time, so that finding what works right now is not necessarily a permanent answer for you.

## ROCHELLE'S STORY

Rochelle came to me in 2004 complaining of weight loss over three months, accompanied by severe abdominal pain. She reported that three months prior, she had developed the onset of a dull pain in the left side of her abdomen. She had been told three years previously that she had diverticulitis, and she had her gallbladder removed. After that, she seemed to be much better. But three weeks before she came to see me, while eating breakfast, she all of a sudden felt very faint. She felt bloated and didn't even want to finish her meal. She rested up for a few days and began to feel a little better.

Several mornings later, again while eating breakfast, Rochelle noticed a pressure in her upper stomach. She became very shaky inside and felt dreadful. Her blood pressure had increased to 190/90, so she went to her local emergency room for evaluation. There she was given an antibiotic for a presumed recurrence of her diverticulitis, despite the fact that her pain and discomfort were caused by a burning sensation in her upper- to mid-stomach area. (Diverticulitis typically involves pain and symptoms in the left lower quadrant of the abdomen.) Blood tests and x-rays were taken but did not clarify the diagnosis.

Rochelle settled down for a few days but then had another episode very similar to the previous ones, with the new onset of loose, watery diarrhea. She was given Lomotil (an anti-diarrheal), and although it did improve her diarrhea, it also set off an increase in abdominal cramping. Rochelle had lost fifteen pounds in only two weeks, and she found that Zantac helped a bit to decrease her stomach pain. When we treated her with Nexium, a somewhat stronger antacid preparation than Zantac, she noted no benefit and continued to experience severe symptoms and lose more weight.

I performed a comprehensive stool analysis and found that Rochelle's body was not digesting fat properly. It also wasn't making enough stomach acid, had low stores of butyrate (a necessary nutrient for colon cells), and most important showed an overgrowth of two different species of Candida. With this information, I started her on betaine hydrochloride to replenish her hydrochloric acid. I also had her take calcium butyrate and digestive enzymes rich in lipase with each meal. I added Diflucan to kill the yeast and placed her on a high-protein, low-carbohydrate diet so that she would not keep feeding the yeast. Carbohydrates are nutrients that feed the yeast (and most of these other toxic microbes), so depriving the yeast of its sustenance is essential to its elimination.

Rochelle responded well to this regimen, and within a month she was markedly improved, with only occasional stomach aches and diarrhea. With the resolution of the abdominal pain, which, in retrospect was clearly caused by irritable bowel syndrome (IBS), we reviewed the concepts of an elimination diet to look for food allergy as a component of her symptoms. We also began the medication Librax, a bowel-calming product. Within a few more weeks Rochelle was completely well. She has continued to do well in the five years since, and as long as she watches her diet and takes her supplements, she is a happy camper.

Rochelle's story is an excellent example of how severe irritable bowel syndrome can be successfully treated by using the concepts discussed in this chapter. The majority of people with this disorder can experience dramatic improvement by looking for intestinal dysbiosis and food allergy and treating them. There is often a stress component to irritable bowel disease, and it helps if we address this as well.

When patients come to my office with unexplained intestinal symptoms and have already had a full evaluation, which usually includes a CT scan of the abdomen and upper and lower endoscopy, most of them can benefit from investigating dysbiosis and food allergy. You might want to reread Olivia's story about food allergies in Chapter 7 to better understand the uses of this treatment process.

## NICK'S STORY

Nick's mother and father brought their nearly two-year-old child to my clinic almost ten years ago. Nick wasn't gaining weight normally and had become very irritable and fussy in his first year of life. Just before I saw him, he had been admitted to a university-based pediatric hospital for three full weeks, diagnosed with pneumonia and what we call "failure to thrive," which simply means that he wasn't growing at a normal rate. Despite intensive evaluation in the hospital and the use of hyperalimentation (a process in which intravenous proteins and lipids are used to help supplement the nutritional process), Nick had still lost another pound. His parents described Nick waking up at night with what seemed to be stomach pain and gas, noting that one night he had awakened and screamed for three hours. As they reflected on his symptoms, his parents were beginning to think that eating cheese may have played a role in his symptoms. (He had been breast-fed for eighteen months and clearly got worse after beginning to consume milk products.)

Nick also had sporadic bouts of diarrhea and frequent episodes of asthma and eczema (a skin rash often associated with allergy). When we checked his stool test, he had a severe overgrowth of Candida and almost no *Lactobacillus* present. So we treated the yeast overgrowth with anti-fungal agents, provided a good supply of probiotics, and took him off all milk products. He began to improve immediately, and slowly, over several years, he moved up the growth chart from below the fifth percentile (meaning really poor growth) to the twenty-fifth percentile, which represents significant improvement. The eczema disappeared, and his asthma improved as well. I have had the opportunity to watch Nick grow into a fine youngster, and his bright eyes and healthy demeanor are a far cry from the sunken skin and dull eyes of his first visit.

In Chapter 9 we will discuss blood sugar and its role in health. Hypoglycemia (low blood sugar) is really about another area of intestinal physiology and fits in nicely with this discussion, so it seems to me that the flow of information should place it next in our narrative. As this will begin Part Two, the section about what I call the "Little Six Health Imbalances," you might wonder why certain discussions merit a "big" designation, while others are "little." Please understand that these names are meant to simplify the process of looking at the complex interweaving of these ideas. The Big Six is just my designation for the six most commonly overlooked components of chronic illness, and the Little Six is my nickname for the six next most common components. It doesn't mean that any one of these is less important than the other (particularly for individuals in which one piece of information may prove pivotal in their cure); it just means that I typically start with the first six because they are statistically the most likely to be a useful starting point for a given patient. We then move into the next grouping if that evaluation does not provide the healing we seek.

So onward to the Little Six.

## FURTHER READING

Crook, William G. M.D., *The Yeast Connection: A Medical Breakthrough*, Vintage Books, 1986.

Truss, Orian C., M.D., *The Missing Diagnosis II*, Birmingham, Alabama, 2009.

# PART TWO

# The "Little Six" Health Imbalances

In Part One I covered a great deal about the most common imbalances that may be contributing to your illness. With a little luck, identifying and treating those imbalances may have cured or greatly improved your health. I sincerely hope that you are now so far along the path of healing that you don't need to dig any deeper. Unfortunately, however, many of my patients—while considerably better and thrilled with their improvement—still need me to delve deeper.

I call the second phase of this "digging deeper" process a search for the Little Six. These are the next most common deficiencies and imbalances that we will pursue. The order in which I do this, as before, depends on the details of my patient's history, and we go after the most likely culprit first.

Part Two starts with assessing a patient for the commonly under-diagnosed condition of low blood sugar, also referred to as hypoglycemia; that is step 1 in our process of looking, in turn, for each of the six less common health imbalances. Then we turn to step 2, the area of dental toxicities, which includes mercury toxicity, imbalances in the electrical charges on different teeth, and root canals. The newly recognized realm of mold toxicity and the larger arena of biotoxicity are covered in step 3. This is followed, in step 4, by the related area of unrecognized chronic infections (which often contribute to biotoxicity) and includes viral and bacterial (especially Lyme disease) species. The importance of looking for chronic infectious diseases cannot be over-emphasized. This chapter is intended as an introduction to this subject that is worthy of its own book. Amino acid deficiencies, particularly because of their importance in building up our neurotransmitters (so important for treating depression and anxiety) are the focus of step 5. Our newest component of this evaluation process, which has added another dimension to our treatments, is that of evaluating and treating methylation defects in step 6.

The vast majority of my patients are much better, often cured, when we have completed these steps. But not everyone gets better. The labels of Big Six and Little Six might imply that once we have completed this process of evaluation, we have looked at everything that can possibly go wrong; alas, this is not so. In Dr. Teitelbaum's book *From Fatigued to Fantastic,* he identifies more than 150 imbalances known to contribute, at times, to the cause(s) of fibromyalgia and chronic fatigue. The good news is that no one has all of these imbalances. However, this information does underscore the fact that there can be a lot more than twelve steps to healing.

It is my hope that I can, in these pages, provide legitimate hope for healing, by explaining, and at times oversimplifying, a complicated process. Medical detectives must be willing to be patient, thoughtful, and diligent in sifting through the clues we have collected to provide a precise diagnosis for our patients. It is through correct diagnosis that we can move toward healing. So please be aware from the beginning of this journey that we may need to keep on digging to find your pay dirt.

When we have completed all of these steps, whether you are better or not, know that there is still much more a knowledgeable and caring physician can do for you.

## CHAPTER 9

# Blood Sugar Imbalances: Hypoglycemia and Insulin Resistance

### Sugar in the Morning, Sugar in the Evening . . .

In the mid-1980s, some people who were inexplicably ill began to learn about a "mythical creature" called *hypoglycemia*. The warnings about this creature were dire: An encounter with it would bring about fatigue, brain fog, difficulty with focus and concentration, shakiness, heart palpitations and sweating, and an overall feeling of discontent. This beast would completely conquer your body, and its presence was explained by the presence of low blood sugar, thus giving it the moniker *hypoglycemia* (*hypo* means low, and *glycemia* refers to sugar in the blood). The science and reality of low blood sugar has been well described in the medical literature. We know that if diabetics take too much insulin or oral medication, their blood sugar can drop to dangerously low levels, so low that they could pass out while walking or driving. We also know that some newborns are particularly prone to low blood sugars, which is a serious medical condition. In fact, at one point in time, hypoglycemia was defined in medical practice as a blood sugar level of 50 mg/dL or lower. This was accepted as standard medical knowledge for decades.

Soon a sizeable group of people began to realize they had symptoms that seemed to correlate with low blood sugar, and they began to visit primary care physicians by the droves. An odd phenomenon occurred: Physicians were uncomfortable with the vague nature of these complaints and what they perceived to be an overall difficulty in managing these patients. There was a clear overlap of these symptoms with anxiety. Heart palpitations and tremor, which are frequent components of hypoglycemia, are often reported as symptoms of anxiety. Many primary care physicians were uncomfortable treating anxiety, preferring to refer those patients to psychiatrists.

In a rather perverse attempt to alleviate physician discomfort—at a great disservice to patients everywhere—several papers were published by endocrinologists in which hypoglycemia was renamed *reactive hypoglycemia*. The implication of this new name was that the presence of a low blood sugar was taken to represent some kind of laboratory glitch that didn't represent a true biochemical event. Hence, the presence of a measured low level of blood sugar could be dismissed out of hand as unimportant or irrelevant. This was wonderful news for many physicians who could then inform their patients that they only had reactive hypoglycemia, which had no medical significance and needed no treatment.

Unfortunately, it also dismissed, out of hand, the presence of very real (not imaginary) low blood sugars that were significantly affecting the health of many individuals. These patients were told that they should seek psychotherapy for what was actually a physical problem.

In other words, patients were informed that these symptoms were to be ignored and were to be labeled as *psychosomatic*. Now this is an interesting word. All it really means is that the mind (*psyche*) and the

### Symptoms of Hypoglycemia
The most significant symptoms of hypoglycemia are:
- Fatigue
- Weakness
- "Brain fog" (inability to think clearly)
- Tachycardia (rapid pulse rate)
- Diaphoresis (sweating)
- Shakiness and tremor
- Anxiety
- Syncope (passing out, when hypoglycemia is severe)

body (*soma*) are one. If something occurs in the body—say, low blood sugar—it affects the mind by directly causing fatigue and difficulty in mental functioning. This is a clear description of what happens to us physiologically, not psychologically. Unfortunately, the meaning of *psychosomatic* has shifted to something it was never intended to convey: that the symptoms are not real and exist only in the mind. That is how the diagnosis of hypoglycemia became a myth. With only a little twist of language, the field of medicine summarily dismissed thousands of patients who were struggling with the symptoms of hypoglycemia, and they simultaneously removed any hope of improvement. This is nothing to be proud of, and regrettably, this misunderstanding persists to this day.

My understanding of low blood sugar is fairly simple: If patients have some, or all, of the symptoms of hypoglycemia (see Symptoms of Hypoglycemia), and also have a low blood sugar level drawn at the time they are experiencing these difficulties, then low blood sugar is probably the cause of their symptoms. Even clearer, if we treat it and the symptoms resolve, then as far as I'm concerned, they have this diagnosis and we're correctly treating it. It really is that simple, at least for me and for my patients. No effort to explain it away or dismiss it out of hand makes any sense to me.

The symptoms experienced by each patient depend largely on the actual blood sugar level, and patients vary in their sensitivity to these levels. Some patients are exquisitely sensitive to minor drops in glucose, and others can tolerate it somewhat better. There is actually a spectrum of symptoms, based on blood sugar levels. So with small drops in blood sugar, the patient is likely to experience fatigue, brain fog, and difficulty with focus or concentration. As the blood sugar drops further, their symptoms may proceed to sweating, heart palpitations, and tachycardia (rapid heart rate), and as the blood sugar levels drops even further, to tremors and full-blown anxiety. I suspect that a large number of people diagnosed with panic attacks and anxiety actually have undiagnosed hypoglycemia.

What is really going on here is that the patients with this problem have what I call a "trigger-happy pancreas." What lowers our blood sugar as it starts to rise when we eat a meal is the secretion of insulin by the pancreas. For patients with hypoglycemia, their pancreas produces too much insulin, and it drops the blood sugar well below normal levels. (I will graph this out for you later in this chapter.) Unfortunately, we cannot promise a cure for hypoglycemia, as the tendency to have a hyperreactive pancreas that produces too much insulin is usually a life-long condition. The good news, however, is that we can treat or manage it quite well. In the best of cases, we can prevent the most serious complication of hypoglycemia: diabetes. It would seem logical that if hypoglycemia is produced by an excessive release of insulin from the pancreas, over time this would eventually exhaust or deplete the pancreas's ability to make insulin, resulting in diabetes. This can and does happen in a significant percentage of patients with hypoglycemia. But if we *prevent* the pancreas from being overtaxed, with proper treatment, the chance of developing diabetes can be reduced drastically.

When people arrive in my office complaining of fatigue or exhaustion, especially in relationship to when they eat their meals, I start to pay close attention. They rarely recognize the problem until we bring it to their attention because they usually assume it is coming from something external. I begin asking them about the potential relationship between the timing of their meals and the onset of their symptoms. Do they get sleepy or tired or weak two hours after lunch? If these symptoms persist and these patients begin to feel shaky or sweaty or they experience heart palpitations, do they feel better after they eat? Many patients have learned to consume sugar regularly (especially soft drinks and candy) throughout the day in order to avoid these symptoms of low blood sugar. But they are unwittingly making themselves worse.

## KARL'S STORY

When I first met him, Karl was a thirty-five-year-old engineer who complained of extreme fatigue to the point of depression. In fact, he thought he was depressed and noted that for the previous ten years, he had been unable to motivate himself to build his business. This was somewhat surprising to him since he'd been a go-getter all his life and thought of himself as a high-powered individual. As he began describing his difficulties to me, Karl admitted that he really didn't recognize himself anymore. It was like he was just going through the motions of life in a kind of fog.

I started by conducting some basic lab work on Karl, including DHEA and magnesium tests, both of which returned normal results. I then gave him a five-hour glucose tolerance test. This test measures a patient's blood sugar level every hour for five hours after consuming a measured amount of glucose. (I will discuss this test in more detail soon.) It documented that he had a profoundly low blood sugar that occurred three hours after consuming the glucose load of the test (which is similar to how the body reacts after eating a meal). So I put him on a program that consisted of a high-protein, low-carbohydrate diet, and included the consumption of high-protein, low-carbohydrate snacks two and a half hours after each meal, to help prevent the drop in blood sugar that we knew, now, would occur at three hours after eating a meal. Just three days later, a completely different Karl stepped into my office. He was bright-eyed and bushy-tailed, no longer morose and down, and he told me that his vitality had completely returned. He was no longer depressed, and he was taking on every project in sight with new enthusiasm.

I have followed Karl for the past ten years, and as long as he eats properly, he is highly motivated and successful at his work. Every once in a while, when he gets sloppy about his diet, symptoms recur, and that is a clear message for him to get back to the diet that he knows works so well for him.

Over the years, I have treated hundreds and hundreds of people like Karl. Most, like Karl, are stunned to discover that if they eat correctly, they can feel amazingly better. Years of malaise can simply melt away.

So here's how it works. When I suspect that a patient might be suffering from hypoglycemia, I perform a standard (but rarely done) five-hour glucose tolerance test. A single blood sugar level, taken at only one time of the day, is not adequate to tell us what we need to know. Keep in mind that blood sugars normally fluctuate throughout the day, and at any one moment in time, that lab test merely reflects the levels at *that* precise moment. Patients respond in unique ways to processing glucose, and a low blood sugar can appear anywhere from one to five hours after we begin the test. Some practitioners even use a six-hour test, but I have not found that extra hour helpful, and it unnecessarily prolongs the testing.

The patient visits her local laboratory after eating nothing past midnight the evening before. Consuming water is fine, but no food or coffee should be ingested from midnight until the time the test begins. The lab begins by drawing a blood glucose level while she is fasting, which is used as our baseline level. The patient is then given a drink containing 75 grams of glucose. After consuming this drink, the lab simply measures her blood glucose every hour for the next five hours. From the patient's perspective, this is an annoying and sometimes difficult test, because if she truly has hypoglycemia, she might get weak, shaky, and anxious during the test. However, if the patient does experience those symptoms at the same time that we find a low blood sugar, it becomes a very useful test, as it often provides information we couldn't otherwise obtain. It is not unusual for patients to discover, when we graph the results of their testing, that a great number of their symptoms are finally explained. I will often hear: "Wow, now I understand why I feel so lousy two hours after lunch." Perhaps more important, when patients see their altered physiology in a black-and-white laboratory report, they begin to realize that their symptoms are not psychological.

When we perform this test, the baseline glucose level is typically 90 mg/dL, and a normal person will usually respond to this glucose challenge with a rise in his blood sugar levels to up to 160 mg/dL at one hour, which then drops back down to 90 mg/dL at two hours. Figure 9.1 shows how we look at blood sugar levels over time. The vertical axis represents the level of blood glucose, and the horizontal axis demonstrates time, starting from baseline at "0" and moving up through the five hours of the test.

What's really happening here, as I described previously, is that in response to a rise in blood glucose, the pancreas, registering that rise in glucose, responds by producing just exactly the right amount of insulin to bring the blood glucose back to baseline.

Now let's look at what a hypoglycemic patient's graph might show in Figure 9.2. This figure shows that even with the same baseline, an individual with hypoglycemia has what I have referred to as a "trig-

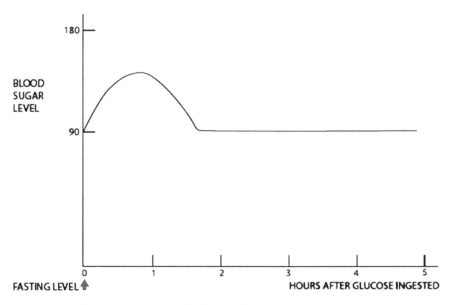

Figure 9.1: Normal 5-Hour Glucose Tolerance Test

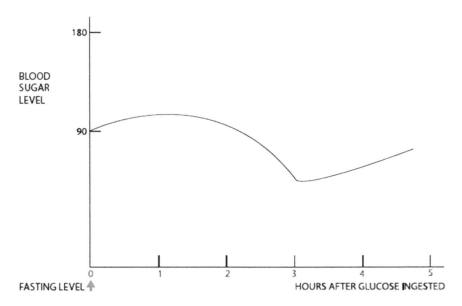

Figure 9.2: 5-Hour Glucose Tolerance Test in Hypoglycemia

ger-happy" pancreas. The pancreas of this hypoglycemic patient, in response to the rising blood sugar level (caused by the carbohydrate provided by a meal) produces too much insulin too soon. This excessive amount of insulin doesn't allow the blood sugar to rise as it normally would. Even more important, the insulin produced in excess by the pancreas causes the blood glucose level to plunge, and it stays down until it can pull itself together and get back to baseline.

Although the medical definition of hypoglycemia is a reading of 50 mg/dL or less, I have found that even blood glucose levels in the 70s can represent true hypoglycemia for some patients. Remember, we are all different biochemically, and some people will become symptomatic at glucose levels that other people may tolerate well. I find that many patients who were labeled "normal" by other doctors really have a treatable condition if they could just get someone to take it seriously. How the patient responds to treatment tells us a great deal. Even the test gives us a great deal of information. If a patient becomes symptomatic at a blood glucose level of 65 mg/dL during the fourth hour of our test, this usually means that when we prevent that drop in blood sugar by our treatment program, they will notice improvement almost immediately. Their tiredness and "brain fog" will clear, and their rapid pulse will become a thing of the past. When a patient improves dramatically with treatment, in my opinion it is presumptive evidence of the accuracy of this diagnosis.

What's happening here is that as the glucose level in the blood drops, the level in the brain also drops. Unlike other body tissues, such as muscle tissue, which can burn any fuel (protein, starch, sugar, or fat), the brain can only utilize or "burn" glucose for energy. If the level of glucose in the brain drops, the brain cannot function properly, leading to the neurological symptoms mentioned earlier that are associated with hypoglycemia.

## Treatment of Hypoglycemia

The treatment of hypoglycemia is essentially threefold. Most important is the institution of a high-protein, low-carbohydrate diet. There are a host of these diets readily available today: Dr. Atkins's, Dr. Galland's, South Beach, Protein Power, Suzanne Somers's, Sugar Buster's, Dr.

Schwarzbein's, Dr. Shoemaker's, and many others. All share the concept of high-protein and low-carbohydrate intake with minor variations between them. How low on carbohydrates? That depends on the individual: Some patients have a fragile system and can only handle 20 grams a day, while others can tolerate between 40 and 60 grams daily. Most will need somewhere between 20 grams and 40 grams for optimal functioning. I hope that the rationale for this diet is obvious: If you don't eat carbohydrates, you don't set off the overreacting pancreatic production of insulin, and hence the blood sugar doesn't fall as dramatically. I usually start with the Atkins diet, as patients find the instructions clear and this diet is quite doable. As patients develop more awareness and knowledge about the relationship of their symptoms to their carbohydrate intake, they may be able to move to the less restrictive diets mentioned above and incorporate the concept of *glycemic index* into their carbohydrate choices.

The glycemic index is a measurement that allows us to compare how much like sugar any other carbohydrate behaves, metabolically, when processed by the body. For example, brown rice has a lower glycemic index than white rice. Berries have a lower glycemic index than bananas. This information allows us to make even better carbohydrate choices.

Secondly, if patients snack on high-protein, low-carbohydrate nutrients (cheese, meats, eggs, nuts, or pork rinds) just before we know their blood sugar will drop, we can also avert the intense drop in blood sugar that sets off symptoms. For example, if the blood glucose drops at three and a half hours on our glucose tolerance test, I would advise a snack timed three hours after every meal to proactively get the jump on that dropping blood sugar.

Lastly, but not as important as dietary interventions, is the use of the mineral chromium, which has been shown to have a mild ability to stabilize blood sugar levels. I typically recommend 200 mcg of chromium picolinate twice a day.

With this program, if a patient indeed has hypoglycemia, the response to our treatment is quite rapid. Within a few days many patients report feeling better than they have in years. As I have emphasized, the response to our treatment actually clarifies the diagnosis because if the patient does not respond to this program, we need to go back to the drawing board to understand what is causing the symptoms. For many of my patients, hypoglycemia is just a part of the problem, but an important part. If over-looked, symptoms may persist despite heroic efforts in other areas.

Hypoglycemia is no myth. It is a commonly overlooked medical con-dition, amenable to treatment, and worth the minor inconvenience of testing to clarify both the diagnosis and treatment.

## INSULIN RESISTANCE

In some respects, insulin resistance is the flip side of hypoglycemia. Here, the body is less sensitive to insulin, and the pancreas has to pro-duce more and more insulin to get the blood sugar to respond properly.

We have come to recognize the importance and frequency of this condition, as the epidemic of obesity in our population has been doc-umented. In fact, insulin resistance is the essence of what has been called metabolic syndrome, syndrome X, or insulin resistance syndrome. This condition has been shown to represent a significant risk factor for coro-nary heart disease, and is associated with a rise in blood sugar, a rise in cholesterol and triglycerides, and a rise in blood pressure, and is recognized as a precursor of full-blown diabetes.

The two most important risk factors connected to this syndrome are the presence of extra weight around the middle and upper part of the body, called central obesity, and insulin resistance.

Too much insulin, which is produced by the body in an attempt to override this resistance, is inflammatory to the body and adds to the burden of inflammation that may already be a difficulty for our chron-ically ill patients.

Adding to this inflammatory process is the metabolism of our fat cells, called adipocytes. For many years, we ignored the fat cells in our body and viewed them as a kind of inert, harmless storage depot that was annoying—for those who put on extra weight—but of no great consequence. However, we have discovered that these fat cells are any-thing but inert. They are metabolically extremely active, producing a host of substances that profoundly affect our chemistry. One of the most important of these is the hormone leptin, whose main role is to tell your brain how much fat you have and to help you know when you have eaten enough food. As we make more fat (as we become more overweight), those fat cells make more inflammatory chemicals, and we try to make more leptin to relieve this inflammation and to get our appetite back under control. This becomes a vicious spiral: The more overweight we become, the more inflamed we become, and the more leptin we make to try to overcome this leptin resistance. Leptin resistance is thus similar to and related to insulin resistance.

While the complicated biochemistry surrounding insulin is beyond the scope of this book, I would like to stress its importance and introduce you to the basic principles of treatment, which happily are similar to the diet that I just proposed for hypoglycemia—hence, its connection to this material.

## Treatment of Insulin (and Leptin) Resistance

At the heart of insulin resistance is the strain put on the pancreas to make more insulin. That strain is created by the carbohydrate content of your diet. When you eat carbohydrates (starches and sugars) your pancreas *must* make insulin in response to that stimulus, and as the cells become more and more resistant to what you are making, the strain becomes greater. This can be measured by a slightly different glucose tolerance test, similar to the one described earlier, but this time lasting only three hours. It also measures *insulin* levels as well as glucose levels at baseline and at thirty minutes, then at one, two, and three hours after ingesting glucose. In this manner we can accurately determine exactly what kind of metabolic pattern we are looking at and orchestrate a clearer treatment program.

The treatment aims, through diet, to decrease the carbohydrate stimulation as much as possible—a process that will vary from person to person. Like the diet for hypoglycemia, the diet for insulin/leptin resistance is high protein and low carbohydrate. The less carbohydrates eaten, the lower the demand on the pancreas for insulin. It is basically that simple.

There is one other physiological consideration that I wish to bring to your attention—and this applies to hypoglycemia as well. We have recently learned that we have receptors on our tongue and in the cells of our small intestine that are responsive to anything sweet. Whenever a sweet substance touches those cells, it sends a signal to the pancreas to make more insulin—in a sense preparing the pancreas for what it thinks is coming down the pike. It does not matter whether that substance is sugar, an artificial sweetener, or a natural sweetener like stevia, agave nectar, or fruit. *Anything* sweet will do this. This means that those who are hoping that non-caloric sweeteners will allow them to assuage their sweet tooth while not gaining weight or calories are making a mistake. Those materials will still stimulate the increase in insulin production that we are trying so hard to avoid, and they must not be consumed by anyone who wishes to address their hypoglycemia or insulin resistance.

The good news is that by carefully evaluating how an individual responds to carbohydrates, we can put together a dietary treatment plan that can bring them back into balance: They will not only feel better, but their risk of developing diabetes and heart disease will be significantly decreased.

## FURTHER READING

Agatson, Arthur, *The South Beach Diet.* New York: Random House, 2003

Atkins, Robert C., *Dr. Atkins New Diet Revolution,* Revised Edition, M. Evans & Company, 2002

Galland, Leo. *The Fat Resistance Diet.* New York: Random House, 2005.

Schwartzbein, Dianna, *The Schwartzbein Principle: The Truth About Losing Weight, Being Healthy and Feeling Younger,* HCI, 1999.

Shoemaker, Ritchie C., *Lose The Weight You Hate!,* Baltimore, MD, Gateway Press, Inc., 2005

Somers, Suzanne, *Suzanne Somers' Eat Great, Lose Weight,* Three Rivers Press, 1999

Steward, Leighton H., et al., *The New Sugar Busters! Cut Sugar to Trim Fat,* Ballantine Books, 2003

CHAPTER 10

# Dental-Related Chronic Illnesses and Heavy-Metal Toxicity

## The Tooth, the Whole Tooth, and Nothing but the Tooth

Why did the Zen Buddhist refuse Novocain when he needed to have his tooth pulled? Because he wanted to *transcend dental medication*. This bad but clever pun will help to launch us into a discussion of dental toxicities.

It is curious that in the field of medicine—especially for family physicians like me who are trained in looking at all systems of the body—two areas of health concern are considered so "specialized" that most physicians know very little about them. Those areas are podiatry (the feet) and dentistry. In all of our medical education, these areas receive short shrift, and we are encouraged to refer every problem in these areas to practitioners of those fields. Consequently, most medical doctors know precious little about the feet or the mouth, and during our medical education and training, we almost get the sense that this information is an unnecessary part of our working knowledge base. This has always seemed a bit strange to me.

Over the past thirty years, largely from the work of pioneering dentist Hal Huggins, however, it has become clear that there are a number of dental problems that can greatly affect the whole body. These include mercury toxicity, electrical effects of the different metals that may be present in the mouth, metal allergy, root canal effects, occult infections, and the effects of dental appliances. Let's delve into each of these areas, but be advised: Most dentists are not aware of much of this information either. In fact, imagine the class-action suits that would occur if the dental profession acknowledged that metal amalgam fillings (with a large percentage of mercury) have been harming us for years. In the current medical/legal climate that won't happen. So if you attempt to discuss this with your dentist, more often than not your dentist will tell you that these concerns are silly or trivial. However, despite that attitude, the fact is that mercury is a seriously toxic metal for the body, even when it is present in only minuscule amounts.

## MERCURY TOXICITY

### Symptoms of Mercury Toxicity

- Cognitive impairment
- Headaches
- Fatigue
- Joint pain
- Peripheral neuropathy (numbness and tingling in the feet and hands)
- Anxiety and/or depression
- Autoimmune diseases
- Metallic taste in the mouth
- Dizziness

We have known about the toxicity of mercury for many years. Calomel, a mercury-containing compound, was used in the eighteenth through nineteenth centuries to treat a wide variety of medical conditions. When used "properly" in those times, calomel gradually made those who used it sicker and sicker, until their hair fell out and they began to salivate uncontrollably. Perversely, these symptoms were taken as a sign that the mercury was beginning to work. It was eventually, albeit slowly, recognized that mercury was truly toxic, and it was removed from the shelves as a dangerous material by the late nineteenth century.

When it was proposed in the 1930s that dental amalgams should utilize mercury as a major ingredient to more easily shape and work dental filling materials, the subject was hotly debated for several years at the American Dental Association's annual meetings. Ultimately, it was decided that the convenience of adding mercury to other metals for the purpose of making dental fillings outweighed the known risks of toxicity. So for the past seventy-five years, the public has been exposed to these dental amalgams, which are usually and erroneously called "silver" fillings. I would venture to say that there are very few mouths in my practice that don't have some of these metal fillings in them, with mercury as a significant component. As time has passed, we have begun to recognize that this process may not have been a wise one. Considering that mercury thermometers are no longer available to the public because of the danger that the mercury represents, and that dentists are required by federal agencies to dispose of their mercury as hazardous waste, it seems strange that the dental profession would be so reluctant to admit that mercury might be dangerous to one's health.

Colorado dentist Hal Huggins has devoted his life to trying to share this information about mercury toxicity. He found that when he removed the fillings of people who were very ill, many of them recovered from a variety of medical conditions, including rheumatoid arthritis and neurological impairments like Parkinson's disease and amyotrophic lateral sclerosis (ALS). Huggins also recognized that mercury *sublimates*, which means that it can move directly from a solid to a gaseous form, without becoming a liquid, just like dry ice. When mercury-containing amalgams are scraped with dental tools, significant amounts of this mercury gas can be released into the body. It can then move directly into body tissues, especially the brain and nerves, where it is bound tightly and directly poisons those tissues. Huggins's pioneering work led, unfortunately, to his persecution and the loss of his dental license in Colorado. He has continued to practice and teach in Mexico. Fortunately, enough open-minded dentists had begun to heed his message and learn his techniques so that this research has continued to grow.

While I suspect that dental amalgams are the major source of mercury toxicity, there are other sources as well. Consumption of certain fish can contribute to mercury toxicity, and there are published lists of which fish should be avoided or limited. For example, there are signs posted in the remote, pristine White Mountains of New Hampshire telling anglers that they should limit their consumption of trout to one per month. For more than twenty years, the health department of the state of Minnesota has published the mercury levels of the different game fish in the state, and this information should be available from almost every state department of health as well. In the food chain, as small fish are eaten by bigger fish, we find the highest levels of mercury in the largest predatory fish, such as shark and swordfish.

We also come into contact with mercury in our environment. A small amount can be inhaled by those who live in close proximity to coal-burning plants, and it has recently been noted that the mercury produced by the coal-burning factories in China ascends into the atmosphere and comes down onto our soil as the prevailing winds blow east across the Pacific Ocean.

Yet another source of mercury is found in vaccinations. Since the 1930s, vaccine manufacturers have used thimerosol, a mercury-containing preservative intended to fight off bacterial contamination. Although it is known that young, developing brains and nervous systems are much more sensitive to mercury and much less able to process or detoxify it, many of our children have been exposed to toxic levels of mercury from this source. Until recently, each thimerosol-containing vaccine has provided up to five parts per million (ppm) of mercury with each injection. This is the upper limit of exposure for mercury (as established by federal standards) for a child. However, the vaccine manufacturers, along with the pediatric profession, have encouraged the "bundling" of vaccines. This entails providing not one vaccine but a whole package of vaccines at one pediatric visit, so that until recently a child might receive up to 125 ppm of mercury at that visit! Many experts have come to suspect that the explosion of autism and attention-deficit hyperactivity disorder (ADHD) may, in part, be directly linked to these vaccinations. Although this connection has been denied, the amount of thimerosol in vaccinations has been sharply reduced in the past few years.

The impetus for this reduction is partly due to the influence of several physicians prominent in this area, most notably Stephanie Cave, M.D., who has published widely and spoken before Congress repeatedly, pleading that thimerosol be removed from these vaccines. In response to this call for action, vaccine manufacturers have minimized (but not completely eliminated) the amount of thimerosol in most vaccines. Concerned parents should really check into their children's vaccinations to be sure they are safe. Flu shots, for example, still contain thimerosol, yet medical authorities now strongly encourage the use of that vaccine in small children. By countering the negative effects of mercury, pioneering physicians in the field of autism have helped many children recover or improve. (We will discuss this part of a comprehensive treatment program for autism in more detail in Chapter 22.)

Germany and Canada have discouraged the use of mercury amalgams. England has taken this problem so seriously that several years ago the country passed a law that requires that the mercury amalgam fillings of the deceased who await cremation be removed prior to cremation so that mercury vapor will not be released into the atmosphere.

If you need to have a filling replaced, please do not allow your dentist to use a mercury-containing, silver-colored amalgam. There are many viable alternatives to using mercury-based fillings. However, merely switching to plastic-based fillings may not be much healthier. One of the more common plastic replacement materials contains a great deal of bisphenol-A, a toxic chemical that can do just as much harm as the mercury. Should you need your fillings replaced, I would strongly advise that you look for a *biological* or *holistic* dentist specifically trained in using alternate dental-filling materials. Testing is available that allows us to know which potential plastic fillings would be best tolerated by an individual. But a word of warning: It has been my patients' experience that when they bring this up for discussion with their regular dentist, they are usually told, "There is more mercury in a can of tuna fish than there is in your mouth." Not only is this untrue, but keep in mind that when the dentist works on the fillings already present in your mouth, scraping them will release mercury vapors, which will add to whatever mercury burden is already present in your body.

## Evaluating Mercury Toxicity

The only diagnostic tool we initially had to evaluate for mercury toxicity was hair analysis. I can't count how many patients whose hair I tested who had false-negative results. It turns out that there are several problems with hair analysis, especially when testing for mercury. First, mercury tends to bind more tightly to other body tissues—so much so that if it is present in the body, we will not find it with simple tests of hair, urine, blood, or stool. That's not where it's present. Mercury tends to bind preferentially to nerve tissue: brain and neurons especially. Second, the results of hair analysis have always been difficult to reproduce. This means that if you cut some hair from your head, separate it into three different batches, and send those to the same laboratory, it is likely that the results will be quite different in all three specimens. This lack of reproducibility has always cast a shadow over laboratory results, and I have found the results of hair analysis to be inaccurate to the point that I don't use it anymore.

So how *do* we check for mercury toxicity? Since it binds so tightly to body tissues, what we need to do is use a chelating material (a chemical binding agent) to bind tighter to the mercury than your body tissues do, and then we can pull the chelated (bound) mercury out into the urine. If there is a significant amount of mercury in a patient's tissues, we will find significant amounts of mercury in his urine as well.

The chelating procedure goes as follows: A patient receives a brief, fifteen-minute intravenous infusion with DMPS, a chemical that binds tightly to mercury (with the rather long and awkward name of 2,3-Dimercapto-1-propanesulfonic acid). The patient then collects all of her urine for a timed period of six to twenty-four hours, and this is mailed to a laboratory that can measure toxicity of heavy metals, of which mercury is a prime example. This is an accurate and elegant test. The amount of mercury measured in the urine is a clear measure of the amount of mercury present in the body, and hence an accurate measure of the mercury toxicity present in the patient.

As a result of this testing process, we can also learn about the presence of other heavy metal toxins: lead, aluminum, nickel, cadmium, arsenic, and others. If we find it, we can treat it, and the removal of other heavy metal toxins may be an important part of our treatment program. While the details of this testing and treatment process may vary from one clinician to another, this discussion represents an accurate consensus. For those patients, especially children, for whom we would prefer not using an intravenous procedure to deliver the binding or chelating chemical, we can use an oral chelating material called DMSA (meso-2,3,-dimercaptosuccinic acid). It is not as strong as DMPS in its ability to pull mercury out of the tissues, but it still allows us to perform the analysis on children safely, without being invasive.

## Treatment for Mercury Toxicity

The treatment for mercury toxicity is similar to the diagnostic proce-dure—that is, we can use regular, monthly intravenous infusions of DMPS or regular oral doses of DMSA to pull mercury out of the body. A note: Chelating agents are utilized for their ability to preferentially bind to heavy metal toxins, but to a small extent they will also bind to some of the essential minerals we need for good health and pull them out of the body, too. Therefore, patients should supplement chelation treatments with oral minerals that include trace minerals. When we refer to minerals, we generally mean the ones that are present in the body in the largest amounts, such as calcium, magnesium, and zinc. "Trace" minerals refers to those minerals that are important but present in only tiny amounts, such as chromium, manganese, molybdenum, selenium, boron, and vanadium. The point that I am trying to make here is that minerals should not be taken on the day of, or the day after, chelation treatments. We don't want the binding properties of the chela-tor to remove the *good* minerals, and we don't want to waste the chela-tion effects by binding the good minerals in lieu of the heavy metal toxins. During chelation, it is also helpful to add some weaker, natural chelating materials, such as vitamin C, chlorella, alpha-lipoic acid, and garlic, to the treatment. By themselves, these supplements will not remove adequate amounts of heavy metal toxins, but when combined with the stronger chelators such as DMPS or DMSA, they will enable those chelators to be more effective, and to help remove from the body those heavy metals as they get mobilized by treatment. Those who are interested in chelation-related diagnosis and treatment should seek help from physicians trained in the chelation process. The American College of Advancement in Medicine (ACAM) and the International College of Integrative Medicine (ICIM) train physicians in the correct use of these materials; and contact them for a list of physicians in your area who do these procedures properly.

Several years ago, a forty-year-old gentleman presented to me with the sudden onset of rheumatoid arthritis. He was working in a difficult environment, several states distant from our office, and for financial reasons, he really needed to keep working at his job but could barely do so. I scrutinized his health history and could not quite understand the sudden onset of his arthritis until I asked about recent dental work. Yes, just two weeks before the onset of his arthritis, he had had extensive dental work done. When I did the DMPS test on him, not only did it show the highest mercury level of any patient we'd ever measured, but he experienced marked relief of his joint pains for the next three days—*simply* from the DMPS chelator used in his test, which pulled a small fraction of mercury out of his body! Unfortunately, as he worked a long distance from our office, and because his family was not supportive of this form of treatment, he pursued more conventional methods of treatment and was lost to follow-up.

I suspect that if we could have removed all of the mercury from his body, he would have done well. It is my experience that rheumatoid arthritis and other autoimmune diseases (such as multiple sclerosis, lupus erythematosus, and scleroderma), chronic fatigue, fibromyalgia, autism, ADHD, and a variety of neurological impairments (such as Parkinson's disease, memory loss, and other cognitive difficulties) are often linked to mercury toxicity. Many other physicians have made similar observations. One of the tip-offs in a patient's history that suggests that mercury may be part of the problem is the sudden onset of memory loss. A patient presented to our office several years ago with just such a problem (see Ed's Story).

## ED'S STORY

Ed was a million-dollar-a-year realtor, very sharp and focused in all of his work activities. But all of a sudden, his memory began to fail him; he couldn't think clearly or even remember his own phone number. He simultaneously developed the onset of fatigue and headaches. He was very frustrated and worried by this sudden turn of events, and visits to several physicians' offices had provided no answers. On our initial testing for Ed, along with having a DHEA deficiency, he had significant levels of mercury in his urine on DMPS testing. With a mouth full of old "silver" amalgam fillings, I felt his symptoms were most likely caused by mercury toxicity. So we treated him with DHEA, 50 mg each morning, and intravenous DMPS on a monthly basis. We also referred him to a biological dentist for proper removal of his amalgam fillings. DMPS typically pulls 1 ng/DL of mercury out of the body per treatment, so the number of treatments usually depends simply on the initial level of mercury, which we obtain at our first analysis.

After six months of treatment, Ed had greatly improved, and within a year he was back at work at full capacity. Not only could he think clearly again, but his headaches and fatigue had also disappeared. This improvement from the treatment for mercury toxicity is a fairly typical occurrence in our office, and it underscores the importance of looking for this diagnosis when the appropriate symptoms are present.

## DENTAL-RELATED ELECTRICAL IMBALANCES

In addition to potential mercury toxicity, metal amalgam fillings may have yet another component of toxicity: the *imbalanced or abnormal electrical potential of the teeth*. This jaw-breaking phrase (sorry about the pun) actually represents a simple concept. Whenever various metals are in close proximity, they essentially create a battery, which produces an electrical charge. Now consider the fact that when your teeth are filled, your dentist, even when he works with the same equipment and mixture of materials, cannot create the exact same *balance* of metals in each amalgam filling. Each filling, therefore, is different in terms of the exact proportion of metals combined in it. If you have a silver amalgam filling next to a gold filling—or a stainless steel crown, or metal beneath the crown placement, or a metallic plate or bridge—you have the presence of multiple metals in close proximity, and this may create a significant electrical charge around each tooth.

The presence of these electrical charges can be easily measured. Dentists trained in this discipline can simply place a probe against each tooth and individually measure the electrical charge. If a significant negative charge is present, this individual's mouth essentially has a battery in it—located mere inches from the base of their brain. It's not much of a stretch to think that this "battery" could short-circuit some of the brain's electrical activity. Unfortunately, the majority of dentists are not yet aware of this information, so they do not have the equipment in their office to take these measurements. If you are concerned about this, seek a dental professional with the knowledge and equipment to evaluate your problem.

Ten years ago, a fifty-year-old gentleman presented to our office with severe tinnitus (ringing in the ears.) The ringing was so loud, so constant, and so insistent that he had become depressed and nonfunctional, and he was awarded disability from Social Security (which is not easy to come by these days). Worse, his depression had grown so intense that he had become suicidal, as he felt he could no longer continue to live with this constant assault on his nervous system. We had the electrical potential of his teeth tested, and the results showed markedly abnormal electrical charges in his largely amalgam-filled mouth. When the dentist we referred him to removed the first few amalgams, his tinnitus was markedly reduced; by the time the fillings were all replaced, his tinnitus was completely gone. He was a most grateful patient, but it is not likely that he would have improved had we not taken this imbalance into consideration.

## ROOT-CANAL TOXICITY

Root canals are another potential cause of dental toxicity. George Meinig, DDS, president of the Root Canal Society and in dentistry for years, came to the sudden realization that he had contributed to making many of his patients sick. He wrote a most courageous book: *Root Canal Cover-Up Exposed!* Dr. Meinig noted that when a root canal procedure is performed, the nerve to the root of the tooth is destroyed. As it turns out, nerves have "trophic" influences on the tissues they supply, meaning that nerves actually nourish and contribute to the blood supply of the surrounding tissues. When the nerve is killed, the blood supply of these tissues is compromised, and this makes them prone to infection. As infection occurs in these dental tissues, the toxins released from the infective agents may cause a variety of medical illnesses. We will discuss this later in this chapter in the section on osteonecrosis. Some holistic dentists who have studied Dr. Meinig's work and used the principles in their own practices have found that their patients' health improves remarkably when the root canal is removed and replaced with a bridge. Since I am not a dentist and do not treat root canals, Michael Rehme, DDS, a holistic dentist from St. Louis, Missouri, has graciously provided me with this clinical example, which we have left unedited, in the patient's own words.

## PATRICK'S STORY

I am a forty-nine-year-old doctor who was in great health. In February 2002, I went for a routine dental visit. I had no symptoms; it was a checkup. X-ray films suggested that an older root canal procedure needed to be redone. An endodontist agreed, and the appointment was scheduled and then performed. I had no problem with the procedure and felt fine after it was completed. Within two days I started to have problems. My blood pressure increased more than twenty points, both systolic and diastolic; within two days of the procedure I developed right and left shoulder pain. This continued and increased over the next eight months. It affected my ability to abduct (lift) my arm—it reminded me of an earlier injury to my shoulder that I had in my early twenties (this happened to be the same time that I had the original root canal done but did not make an impression until now). The reflex for the tooth, according to the tooth chart, showed that it referred to the shoulders. Within a few days my resting pulse and my working pulse and my exercising pulse increased by about ten beats per minute. This did not improve.

As a doctor, I measure different people's grip strength. Before the root canal [my grip strength] averaged 220 pounds; within two days it dropped to 160 pounds. It slowly returned to 180 pounds. Shortly after the root canal, I developed a chronic athlete's foot condition over my foot reflexology point for the shoulder. Within a few months I was starting to feel some brain fog. (I was forty-nine years old!)

After reading several books on root canal problems, I knew that I had to remove the tooth, which had continued to feel nonsymptomatic. My dentist extracted the tooth.

Within two days, my grip returned to 220 pounds, 85 percent of my shoulder pain was gone, my foot infection was gone, brain fog was gone, pulses returned to normal . . . all of my problems were gone with the exception of the blood pressure; it is improving more slowly than I would like, [but] it is getting closer to older readings. I am glad that I removed the root canal tooth. I now wish that I did not wait eight months.

## METAL ALLERGY TOXICITY

One relatively rare cause of dental problems is that of metal allergy. An allergy to nickel, however, is not uncommon, and nickel is often used in stainless steel and other dental appliances. Occasionally, we find patients actually allergic to mercury or gold, in which case the fillings themselves may be causing an ongoing reaction that the patient cannot cure unless the fillings are removed.

One young woman I treated was a dentist who had been wrestling with chronic fatigue and fibromyalgia, and she turned out to be allergic to gold. And, of course, she had multiple gold fillings. She even noticed that when she wore gold jewelry she developed a rash and a worsening of her symptoms, but she was hesitant to admit to herself that her favorite jewelry was contributing to her illness. When we tested her blood with the ELISA/ACT test (see Chapter 7), it was clear that gold was the problem. She reluctantly realized she would have to stop wearing her gold jewelry and get her gold fillings replaced.

## TOXICITIES RELATED TO DENTAL APPLIANCES

Other possible dental sources that may contribute to health impairments can be found in the form of appliances placed into the mouth. I have had a number of patients who developed sudden onset of seizures following the tightening of newly applied braces. Other patients have had exacerbations of their headaches (especially migraines) or sudden onset of tinnitus and ear pain when their braces were tightened or spacers expanded. One young man, aged eighteen, who had had his braces tightened, was treated by his neurologist for seizures for months with poor control. This means that despite the use of a great deal of medication, which left him numb and sleepy and made it hard for him to function, he was still having regular seizures. I treated him with osteopathic cranial manipulation to undo the effects of the tightened braces, but the seizures did not fully resolve until his braces were removed. The orthodontist who applied the braces insisted that it was not possible that the tightening of his braces caused these problems, but improvement did not occur fully until the braces were removed. Interestingly, each time the braces were tightened, the seizures got worse for this patient. Similarly, I have had several teenagers whose migraine headaches got much worse every time their braces were tightened. We will discuss the treatment aspects of cranial manipulation in more detail in Chapter 17.

## OSTEONECROSIS: OCCULT INFECTIONS IN THE JAW

Yet another dental issue that is receiving quite a bit of attention now is that of occult infection found in the jaw. This is given the common name of *cavitations,* or more specifically *osteonecrosis* (from "osteo," meaning "bone," and "necrosis," meaning "destruction of"). This condition is difficult to diagnose with ordinary dental x-rays; it requires an ICAT (a three-dimensional CT scan) to be able to visualize it. Hidden pockets, or cavities, with smoldering infection can persist for years, and unless a dental specialist can open up those pockets and drain the infection, these infections may contribute to chronic illness without our having any awareness of them.

Please understand: I am not suggesting that everyone run out and have all of their amalgam fillings or root canals removed. This process would involve considerable expense and pain, and the inappropriate removal of amalgam fillings could make some individuals worse. If the removal of your amalgams is even a consideration, first get your mercury levels measured and have the electrical potential of your teeth checked. If these tests are negative, there is little reason to pursue the removal of your fillings.

If we do find elevated levels of mercury in an otherwise healthy individual (which we do find, on occasion), what does this mean? I believe that if a patient is basically healthy, her body can "throw off" or handle the negative effects of that toxicity. However, if that same patient gets sick, or is exposed to additional toxins or severe stress, she may become overwhelmed by cumulative toxicity. Now her toxic level of mercury comes into play as an additional weakening factor, which may make it more difficult for her to heal. She has become not only sick, but mercury-toxic as well. We see this component in some of our sickest individuals with Lyme disease, in which the mercury toxicity affects their abilities to remove the toxins produced in their bodies when we are actively killing the Lyme bacteria.

When my wife and I measured our own mercury levels, we discovered they were quite elevated. We both underwent DMPS intravenous therapy to remove the mercury from our bodies. We felt there was no reason to wait around for something bad to happen. Preventive medicine clearly has its place, and this is one example.

You can see that the subject of dentistry is indeed important to your health. It is my intention to provide helpful directions to explore, but I cannot hope to cover all of dentistry within this book. Finding a good holistic dentist may be the first step in this segment of your journey. (Visit www.iaomt.org for a listing of holistic dentists in your area.)

## FURTHER READING

Cave, Stephanie, and Deborah Mitchell. *What Your Doctor May Not Tell You About Children's Vaccinations.* New York: Grand Central Publishing, 2001. This book is an updated and excellent discussion of vaccine safety and usage.

Huggins, Hal A. *It's All in Your Head: The Link Between Mercury Amalgams and Illness.* Garden City Park, NY: Avery Publishing, 1993. This book provides a wonderful overview of mercury fillings and toxicity.

International Academy of Oral Medicine and Toxicology at http://iaomt.org. This site includes information about biological dentistry and will help you find a knowledgeable holistic dentist in your area.

Meinig, George E. *Root Canal Cover-up Exposed!* Ojai, CA: Bion Publishing, 1993. This book includes an in-depth discussion of the problems following root canal procedures.

Seafood Watch Program. Monterey Bay Aquarium Foundation at www.seafoodwatch.org. This site provides comprehensive information about the mercury content of seafood and makes recommendations for consumption.

# CHAPTER 11

# Mold-Related Illness and Biotoxicity

---

## There's a Fungus Among Us

When it comes to understanding the different components of chronic illness, the concept of mold toxicity has received a good deal of recent attention. With the publication of Dr. Ritchie Shoemaker's brilliant books *Mold Warriors* (*2005*) and *Surviving Mold* (*2011*), we now have some tools to both evaluate and treat mold toxicity in its different forms.

A toxin is simply a poison. Microbes (bacteria, viruses, fungi, parasites, or other infective agents) in our body infect us and produce poisons that make us sick—a phenomenon referred to as biotoxicity. Treating disease-causing microbes with medications and other methods will usually make us better. That part of the infection/treatment process is fairly obvious and straightforward. What is just becoming clear to us, however, is that not only do these microbes make us sick by causing an infection, some of them—in the process of being killed by our immune system—can release *more* toxins into our bodies that make us even sicker. Because these toxins are made by microbes, which are living biological systems, we call them biotoxins. (This term distinguishes microbe-related toxins from other types of toxins, such as heavy metal toxins or synthetic toxins, which are not made by living systems.)

Doctors are beginning to understand that some of these toxins remain in the body and cannot easily be excreted or destroyed. Thus, they actually accumulate within our bodies. The body's natural method for processing biotoxins is to concentrate them in the body's main organ of detoxification: the liver. Once the biotoxins congregate in the liver, they bind to the body's bile (produced by the gallbladder) and are sent out into the gastrointestinal tract for release in the stool. However, as the liver binds the toxin to bile and sends it into the intestines, the body's natural recycling system, which is called *enterohepatic circulation*, recirculates the bile when it reaches the small intestine. So the toxin, still attached to that bile secreted by the gallbladder, goes back to the liver rather than leaving the intestinal system. That is how it accumulates within our body. Hence, even when we kill the invading microbes with our immune system, the remaining toxins continue to plague us with their harmful effects. Not everyone is subject to this problem, however. For most of us, the immune system recognizes these toxins and uses its defense mechanisms to destroy them. Unfortunately, about 25 percent of people are genetically unable to make an antibody to these toxins, and those patients may get progressively sicker as the toxins accumulate within their bodies.

What specific microbes are we talking about? The most common offenders are molds, especially the black mold *Stachybotrys.* and *Aspergillus.* But several other mold genuses, such as *Chaetomium, Penicillium, Walleria,* and *Fusarium* can play a role in toxin formation. Harmful toxins can also be produced by certain viruses, especially those in the herpes family, such as Epstein-Barr virus (which is the agent of mononucleosis); cytomegalovirus; and human herpes virus 6 (HHV6), which is the agent of roseola infection. A new and particularly toxic strain of HHV6 has recently been discovered and has now been linked to chronic fatigue and fibromyalgia. Lyme bacteria and the co-infections that accompany Lyme disease (*Bartonella, Babesia,* and *Ehrlichia* — see Chapter 12), can also produce these toxins, as can infections with the mycoplasmas and *Chlamydia pneumoniae,* which are infective particles between viruses and bacteria in size. The atypical pneumonias (walking pneumonia) present examples of these infective agents.

Dr. Ritchie Shoemaker is the physician who first demonstrated the presence of toxins in our environment with his pioneering work on the 1997 *Pfiesteria* outbreak associated with large fish kills in Chesapeake Bay. He later found similar microbes in algae-borne lakes in Florida and in long-standing cases of ciguatera poisoning (which occurs from

eating certain seafood). We suspect that other microbes will be implicated as our understanding of this problem deepens.

## Symptoms of Biotoxicity

So what are the symptoms of biotoxicity? People with this problem may
experience a surprisingly wide range of symptoms related to many different organ systems (see Common Symptoms of Biotoxicity). When

---

### Common Symptoms of Biotoxicity

- Fatigue
- Muscle aches and cramps
- Unusual pains ("ice pick" or "lightning bolt" sensations)
- Sensitivity to bright light, tearing, blurred vision
- Cough, chest pain, shortness of breath
- Cognitive impairment
- Appetite swings and weight gain
- Numbness and tingling, often in unusual patterns
- Frequent urination
- Sensitivity to static electrical shocks
- Excessive thirst
- Menorrhagia (abnormal vaginal bleeding)
- Weakness
- Headaches
- Abdominal pain, nausea, diarrhea
- Chronic sinus congestion
- Joint pain with morning stiffness
- Skin sensitivity to light touch
- Mood swings

---

this confusing array of symptoms is taken out of context or not understood as representing the many manifestations of biotoxicity, it is easy
to see how both patients and physicians might mistakenly think that
this is all "in their heads."

In adults, the symptoms of biotoxicity are very similar to those of fibromyalgia, chronic fatigue, or depression. In children, these symptoms might appear as attention-deficit hyperactivity disorder (ADHD). In fact, many patients with these diagnoses may have unrecognized biotoxicity as either a component of their illness or the direct cause, and most of them would benefit greatly from an evaluation for mold toxicity and treatment if appropriate.

## Diagnosis of Biotoxicity

The first order of business is to even *consider* the diagnosis of mold toxicity. Until I had read Dr. Shoemaker's books and studied with him, I had never thought to ask my patients about their exposure to mold or similar infective agents. Now I routinely inquire about their possible exposure to mold at home or work. Have their homes had any water damage or leakage anywhere? This includes the roof, basement, crawl space, and walls. Do they notice a musty smell or see any mold? The materials that can be seen are often just the tip of the iceberg. Mold may grow inside of walls and get into the heating-cooling system of the house, sending mold spores over the entire residence. If you are wondering how this happens, be aware that Sheetrock paper is made from processed tree bark, which is loaded with mold spores. To bring those spores to life, just add water. How about at work? Do coworkers have similar symptoms or complaints? As I have explored this area, I have been surprised by how many of my sick patients do report exposures to these toxins, because they had never suspected them as being relevant to their illness. Keep in mind that mold toxin may remain in the body for long periods of time, so that mold exposure may have occurred in a previous residence—and I therefore have to ask about *any* exposures—and the toxin may still be present in their body, even though they left that home several years ago.

When presented with this information, some physicians dismiss the whole subject by pointing out that in the natural world we are literally surrounded by molds, so why are we making such a big deal out of this? It is certainly true that our natural world is filled with molds—thousands of species, actually—of every shape and description. In fact, the reason that the mold species make toxins is not to damage us, but to keep other species of mold at bay as the molds try to claim their own piece of real estate in the natural world. It is a system of checks and balances, with each species holding the ones nearby at arm's (spore's) reach. However, when a species of mold can grow inside of a dampened wall with no natural competition, it just grows wild and can make significantly more toxins and many more spores as it reproduces at will. While most mold genuses and their species are relatively harmless to humans, several of them, including *Stachybotrys, Penicillium, Chaetomium, Walleria,* and *Aspergillus,* are capable of producing a toxin that can make us quite ill. Two *Stachybotrys* species—*Stachybotrys chartarum* (*S. chartarum*) and *Stachybotrys chlorohalonata* (*S. chlorohalonata*)—also known as black mold, are the most well known of these.

We can test for the presence of mold in a home with a wide variety of techniques. While not precise, an inexpensive and simple method is to open a mold plate (a Petri dish with a medium that preferentially grows mold) in a questionable room and leave it open for two hours, then replace the top. If a lot of mold is clearly growing on that plate, that growth can be analyzed for the exact mold species present in the room and an estimate of its severity provided. The best and most accurate measurement, according to Dr. Shoemaker, is the ERMI test (ERMI stands for environmental relative moldiness index), in which 5 gm of dust is carefully vacuumed and sent in for analysis. Patients who are reluctant to consider the possibility of mold toxicity are often convinced when they can see laboratory evidence of significant mold growth.

## MAUREEN'S STORY

Maureen was a twenty-eight-year-old woman whom I saw for the first time in March 2006. Her symptoms had begun three years previously, when she was working in a building with a very leaky roof. She had also experienced several traumatic events at the same time, including a difficult divorce, which complicated both our evaluation and her perceptions about what may have triggered her illness. In August 2005, Maureen began to violently throw up on a daily basis, and this went on for months. She saw multiple physicians, including several gastrointestinal specialists, and underwent extensive testing that showed no obvious cause for her symptoms. She was diagnosed by various physicians as having bipolar disorder, irritable bowel syndrome, and hypochondriasis (meaning it was all in her head or psychosomatic). Since her initial exposure to the mold, Maureen had gained thirty-five pounds and had developed sensitivities to all sorts of chemicals and perfumes (which we call multiple chemical sensitivity). This is actually a common event following untreated biotoxin exposure. She continued to experience daily nausea and vomiting, regular headaches, and an inability to think clearly. She described her poor decision making in very simple terms: "It's like I'm inept." She also reported blurred vision and bouts of chest tightness with wheezing.

When Maureen came to see me, she had just lost her job of fourteen years, at which she had been previously quite competent, and she was trying to live a normal life and raise her three children. But she could hardly function. Her energy level was very low, and she reported difficulty in staying asleep and woke up unrefreshed each morning. She described joint pains in her neck, shoulders, and upper back, and she displayed the classic irritable bowel symptoms of gas, bloating, distention, and diarrhea alternating with constipation.

When I tested her vision with the functional acuity contrast test (FACT), which I will describe later, the results strongly suggested biotoxin exposure. Her DHEA test was a little low, as was her progesterone level. I started her on natural progesterone cream, a quarter teaspoon daily, applied to her skin. I also put her on a small dose of DHEA, and we started cholestyramine in the form of Questran, one scoop mixed with water three times daily, which is the best immediate treatment for mold toxicity.

When Maureen returned in April, just six weeks later, she reported that she was already 80 percent better. Her energy was markedly improved despite the fact that she was still living in her home, which had obvious mold growth. She had a new job, was successfully working again, but noticed when she missed even a single day of her Questran that she became lethargic again. She planned to remediate her home to clean up the mold, and she was thrilled that she had her life back; she was no longer plagued by nausea and vomiting, chest pain, and joint pain.

She was so impressed with her improvement in just a short period of time, that she bought a copy of *Mold Warriors* to give to her family physician, who had essentially told her she was a hypochondriac. Her physician refused to even look at the book or to take Maureen's story seriously.

---

It has been my experience that most of our mold-toxic patients have had a similar experience to Maureen's. Their symptoms are usually misunderstood as representing psychological imbalances, particularly depression or anxiety, but they do not respond well to antidepressants and anti-anxiety medications. That should be the tip-off that we need to look deeper for a cause of these symptoms. Recalling that since 25 percent of patients are genetically unable to make the antibodies they need to destroy these toxins, these patients may live in a home with others who have no symptoms or work in a mold-laden environment where others are not sick. Family and coworkers therefore assume that since only one person is sick that it is in that person's head. These people feel like no one is listening to them, including their physicians. The truth is that no one *is* listening. This adds even more to their burden of suffering, often tearing up families and friendships, making them even sicker. Now they are sick *and* depressed, but we can clearly see which came first. It is difficult to try to fight a biotoxin illness, and even more difficult when no one really believes you are sick.

The good news, however, is that we are now beginning to understand these symptoms, and there are treatments available. Newly available testing allows us to measure the presence of mycotoxin in the body, and we can demonstrate the effects of toxins in several ways.

The simplest and most inexpensive test is a visual screening test called the *functional acuity contrast test* (FACT) or the visual contrast test (VCS test). This is a well-established analysis used by ophthalmologists for many years, in which the patient looks at a series of gray and white lines that change in terms of clarity and image and fineness of line. If the patient is unable to see the lighter lines that normal people can, this indicates poor retinal function and has been closely linked to biotoxicity. Maureen was unable to see any of the lines on the last two of five columns, which is strongly indicative of biotoxin illness. You can go to Dr. Shoemaker's website to take this test online (www.survivingmold .com/store1/online-screening-test).

Dr. Hooper at RealTime Laboratories now provides a urine test for three specific mycotoxins: Ochratoxin A, Aflatoxins, and Trichothecenes, which is extremely helpful in enabling us to clarify this diagnosis and to follow treatments.

Dr. Shoemaker has discovered a whole series of biochemical tests that show the patient is experiencing an inflammatory reaction to toxin. He has clearly demonstrated that a untreated patient, when placed in a moldy environment, will have noticeably elevated levels of these inflammatory markers (measured in blood tests), which then come back to normal when the patient is removed from the moldy environment and treatment has been resumed. Once the diagnosis of biotoxicity has been tentatively made, we can begin treatment. In fact, the response to treatment confirms the diagnosis, as in Maureen's case. We can also measure the genetic potential of having an impaired ability to deal with mold (or Lyme disease) with a relatively easy-to-measure blood test called an HLA DR.

## Treatment of Biotoxicity/Mold Toxicity

Several treatments for biotoxicity are currently in use. Dr. Shoemaker provides a combination of medications based on his testing. In its simplest form, treatment consists of using the binding resin cholestyramine (trade name Questran) or its cousin Welchol. These prescription medications are more traditionally used in the treatment of elevated cholesterol levels. But for our mold-toxic patients, these medications bind to the toxin more strongly than the toxin binds to bile, and thus these medications pull toxins out of the intestinal tract while the bile returns to the liver. This drastically decreases the body's load of toxin and allows healing to begin. Dr. Shoemaker has also discovered that combining cholestyramine with Actos provides significantly better results. Actos is usually prescribed for the treatment of diabetes, but for the treatment of mold toxicity we term its use as an "off-label" use. Many medications have value for the treatment of conditions other than the ones for which they are typically provided, and the "off-label" use of a medication is common in the practice of medicine.

Dr. Patricia Kane, who is an expert in the field of fatty-acid metabolism, has developed a slightly different and more complex treatment for mold toxicity. This consists of regular intravenous infusions of phosphatidylcholine followed by intravenous glutathione and intravenous sodium butyrate. This is combined with a special diet (similar to Dr. Shoemaker's), which is essentially a high-protein, low-carbohydrate diet that is particularly rich in omega-3 fatty acids, and many supplements. The intravenous agents used are natural materials that have the capacity to bind well to toxins, and Dr. Kane has reported some remarkable results from her treatment, which we have seen in many of our patients as well.

I can confirm that for many seriously ill patients, these treatments do work, and some patients who have been given up on by their physicians as being hopeless or untreatable have been able to resume a normal life.

## BARBARA'S STORY

Barbara had been my patient for almost eight years when she came into my office in 2008 with some new and frightening symptoms. Let me provide a little medical background for Barbara's history.

When I first saw Barbara, she was a thirty-four-year-old nurse who had not been able to work because of debilitating chronic fatigue, complex partial temporal lobe seizures, migraine headaches, and weakness of her right upper arm. Along with administering osteopathic cranial manipulation, which proved very helpful for her migraines and seizures, I also found her to be low in DHEA and magnesium. She had significant hypoglycemia and an overgrowth of the yeast *Candida albicans* and the bacterial pathogen *Klebsiella*. Her Lyme and heavy metal test results were negative. As I treated all of these imbalances, Barbara improved slowly and steadily, with eventual resolution of all of her symptoms. She was able to return to full-time work as a nurse. Over the next eight years, she would have occasional injuries to her neck and back that would throw her off for a few weeks, but these injuries responded well to osteopathic manipulation.

So, Barbara had essentially been quite healthy until the summer of 2008, when she appeared in my office complaining of a recurrence of her seizures, which hadn't happened in years. She was also experiencing severe migraine headaches and neck pain. With slurred speech and glazed eyes, she told me that she'd never felt this bad; she reported that her face felt funny and she was having strange sensations in her head. Barbara had become so weak that she could only walk with a broad-based gait, and she had developed tremors in her right hand.

She also noted extreme heat intolerance and an odd sensation of chest tightness that came and went.

This sudden deterioration of cognitive and nerve function really had Barbara shaken. It had me shaken, too, as she sat before me and I watched as she could barely speak or answer questions. I immediately got an MRI scan of her brain and consulted her neurologist for evaluation. The MRI scan was clear, showing no pathology. Barbara's neurologist was unable to find a cause for these symptoms, so he prescribed her a small dose of Zoloft for depression and anxiety.

With a normal MRI result and no obvious neurological diagnosis, I started looking elsewhere for answers. We tested her vision with the FACT test and it suggested the possibility of biotoxicity. Further questioning revealed that she had noticed a funny smell in her bedroom, possibly mold, and she reported wiping some of the black mold off of her window sill. The smell was similar to the mulch she had placed under the bedroom window. Only one explanation made any sense to me: with her wide array of debilitating symptoms, Barbara was suffering from biotoxicity, most likely from mold exposure. As we explored this possibility together, we discovered that the timing of this exposure fit well with the onset of her unusual symptoms. I placed her on Questran, one scoop daily, and increased the dosage slowly to two or more scoops per day. She quickly started to improve, and within ten days she could think and walk again. Overall, she estimated a 50 percent improvement. Full-blown seizures were now rare, her headaches were lessening, and she could talk without difficulty. The Zoloft was clearly not helping her and only made her sleepy, so she discontinued it with my blessings.

Barbara hired an environmental consultant to check her home for mold, and mold was indeed discovered under her house. Although I advised her to leave the home until it could be remediated, she was unable to do so for logistical reasons and so I added Actos, 45 mg daily, to her regimen. Within twenty-four hours she called me to say she was almost back to normal and was thrilled with her improvement. She admitted she had been terrified about how poorly her mind was working, and the dramatic relief that she experienced was liberating for her. The tremors and seizures had resolved and she was back to being herself again. She still had to address the presence of mold in her home, which was successfully remediated. She will need to be vigilant in the future to avoid exposure to mold. However, Barbara now knows what she is experiencing when these symptoms reappear, and she now has the medications with which to treat them.

You can now see how devastating mold exposure can be, especially since many physicians, even experts, are unfamiliar with it as a diagnosis. It is my opinion that countless individuals suffer from this condition to different degrees. Without a clear awareness of the existence of biotoxicity, doctors treat people with these symptoms with antidepressants and other medications that might, if they are lucky, take the edge off of their symptoms. These medicines, unfortunately, cannot provide the definitive help these patients so desperately need.

Keep in mind that this is *not* an infection or allergy to mold (although these can occur simultaneously, further complicating and confusing the situation). Instead, this condition is a reaction to mold *toxin,* which, in essence, is a new concept for medical science. I have referred elsewhere to the difficulty that medicine has with embracing new concepts, and this is a perfect illustration of how the reluctance to accept new ideas can hinder a patient's ability to obtain correct diagnosis or treatment.

Whenever anyone develops unusual symptoms that do not fit into a clear diagnostic pattern, always consider the possibility of mold toxicity and Lyme disease.

## FURTHER READING

Foster, John, Patricia Kane, and Neal Speight. *The Detoxx Book.* BodyBio, 2002; available from www.detoxxbook.com.

Shoemaker, Ritchie C. *Mold Warriors.* Baltimore, MD: Gateway Press, 2005.

Shoemaker, Ritchie C. *Surviving Mold: Life in the Era of Dangerous Buildings.* Baltimore, MD: Otter Bay Books, 2010.

RealTime Laboratories, Inc., 4100 Fairway Court, Ste 600, Carrolton TX, 75010, Phone: 972-243-7754 www.RealTimeLab.com

For a more detailed discussion of mold toxicity, I invite the reader to go to a two-hour presentation given to the Mendocino Coast Hospital and filmed for public television. Go to www.mcdh.org, then go to Health& Wellness, then click on Videos on Demand.

Medical professionals may obtain the functional acuity contrast test (FACT) at www.survivingmold.com.

# CHAPTER 12

# Chronic Infections

---

## Don't Bug Me Anymore!

That our universe is filled with potentially infectious agents is certain. They include:

- Bacteria
- Viruses
- Rickettsia (life-forms intermediate in size between bacteria and viruses)
- Fungi and molds
- Parasites
- Prions (misfolded proteins that make up infectious agents)

Please keep in mind that each of the categories listed contain hundreds, even thousands, of unique infectious microbes. If one were prone to paranoia, this would be an excellent place to get started. This is well illustrated in the television show *Monk,* in which actor Tony Shalhoub's character is so fastidious that he has difficulty shaking hands without calling immediately for his hand wipes. From the beginning of time, the presence of germs in our environment has been a simple reality that we've just had to accept and respect. There is nothing we can do to change it—like it or not, we share this planet with the microbes. Understandably, some anxious individuals try to control or contain these organisms, but as we will see, that is not a real option. On the other hand, we may not need to control them. Perhaps all we must do is find a way to coexist with them.

The good news is that our immune system is fairly well designed to do just that. When we are exposed to infectious agents, we have an elaborate method for recognizing and dealing with them. Over the eons of human evolution, we've actually developed a very complicated relationship with these organisms, some of which have been very helpful to us and continue to be so. Recent research suggests that as much as 85 percent of our DNA is actually of viral or bacterial origin! This implies that our relationship with these organisms over time has been symbiotic, or mutually beneficial. This perspective may come as a shock to those of you who assume that any infectious agent is, by definition, an enemy. I urge you to keep in mind that old aphorism: "What doesn't kill you makes you stronger."

Simple examples of this symbiotic relationship between our bodies and these organisms are plentiful. For example, the structure of our mitochondria, the little energy-making factories inside of every cell, is amazingly similar to the structure of bacteria. This suggests that somewhere in our evolution we may have co-opted these bacteria and incorporated them into our structure, making them an important part of us. Another example we discussed earlier is that the health and normal functioning of our intestines depend on a good quantity and balance of beneficial bacteria, namely *Lactobacilli* and *Bifidobacteria*. Indeed, these bacteria produce most of our vitamin B12, so we need that relationship for optimal functioning. Recent research goes beyond this simple coexistence between our bodies and microbes. Evidence now suggests that the microorganisms we were born with and acquired immediately after birth literally create a setting for our body's immune system that resonates in us for the rest of our lives. When that setting is disturbed, getting back into a balance that duplicates our original birth pattern is one key to pursuing good health.

Having said that—and in trying to emphasize the biological balance that is so necessary for health—I also want to stress that certain microorganisms, although beneficial under certain circumstances, can still create significant problems when not in proper balance with our immune system; others are outright toxic to us.

## SUPERBUGS

Severe and even fatal infections are headline grabbers. The media often try to educate us about a possible future in which certain of these infections are potentially preeminent. Major among these infections are the *superbugs,* a term that describes what has been happening since we began using antibiotics a bit too casually. The development of penicillin in the 1940s began the discovery of a host of antibiotics that were capable of killing bacteria. Recently, we have added the ability to kill some viruses as well. This is without question one of the great achievements of modern medicine. It has allowed us, for the first time in history, to treat truly severe and life-threatening infections such as meningitis, pneumonia, and septicemia. Unfortunately, our unbridled admiration for antibiotics has led us to use them at times when they are not really necessary. For example, the majority of sinus, bronchial, and ear infections are caused by viruses for which we do not yet have antibiotic treatments available. There has been a huge push in the medical journals over the past ten years to persuade physicians not to use an antibiotic for every one of these infections, a standard practice for the medical field. The reason for this educational effort is simple: We have slowly but surely killed off the weakest bacteria, and the stronger species have evolved biochemical mechanisms to resist our antibiotics. Thus, these bacteria get stronger and stronger with every passing decade. Some experts fear that within the next ten to twenty years, we will have very few effective antibiotics available.

Let me take a moment to clarify the difference between what we generically call an antibiotic and what we call an antiviral or antiparasitic medication. Technically, the word *antibiotic* means "anti" (against) "life" (or life form), so that any medication that kills any organism *could* be called an antibiotic. However, most physicians, me included, think of antibiotics as being specifically directed against bacteria, not all life-forms. What's the difference, you ask? Antibacterial medications, which is what we usually mean when we use the word *antibiotic,* kill the good bacteria in our intestines and upset the vital ecological balance in those tissues. Antiviral materials (or antiparasitics) specifically kill those named microbes, and do not upset the balance. If we use these words properly, we will not confuse our patients about how we are directing our treatments.

Within the superbug category, the media have singled out several for our immediate attention. One is the dreaded methicillin-resistant *Staphylococcus aureus* (MRSA). In fact, the *Staphylococcus* bacterium (abbreviated *Staph*) is one of the most common infectious agents. Impetigo, along with other skin infections like abscesses, wound infections, and cellulitis, as well as conditions like pneumonia, sinus infections, and ear infections, are well known to be frequently caused by *Staphylococcus*. It is against these particular bacteria that our indiscriminate use of antibiotics has surfaced with a vengeance. These bacteria are no longer susceptible to many of the antibiotics commonly in use, and we have to use multiple antibiotics simultaneously and for longer periods of time. When these infections are especially severe, we may require intravenous infusions in a hospital environment to eradicate the infection. In the discussion of intestinal dysbiosis in Chapter 8, I described how the indiscriminate use of antibiotics can kill off good bacteria and leave more toxic bacteria and yeast behind to inflame our intestines and throw off our biochemical balance. The same effect arises from the use of antibiotics to treat any bodily system. When we discuss the treatment of Lyme disease below, notice that effective treatment of Lyme disease may require prolonged treatment with multiple antibiotics or the use of intravenous antibiotics, which is analogous to our treatment of MRSA.

Let's look at several specific bacterial infections that often go unrecognized and can lead to a weakened state and, ultimately, to the onset of chronic illness. There are aspects of these infections that are controversial, which may explain why they are often not recognized or are overlooked by many healthcare providers.

## LYME DISEASE

When we are bitten by ticks, *Borrelia* bacteria may be injected into our bodies, along with other bacteria and parasites. Tick bites, for this reason, are often referred to as "nature's dirty needle." Some physicians believe that this results in a limited illness and that the timely use of antibiotics for ten to fourteen days will eradicate it completely and forever. This is the view of the Infectious Disease Society of America (IDSA), whose guidelines are published in the *Journal of Infectious Dis-*

*eases.* They do not recognize the existence of chronic Lyme disease, but they sometimes refer to a "post–Lyme disease syndrome." The IDSA believes that the classic bull's-eye skin rash associated with Lyme disease and standard lab tests are quite reliable to make a Lyme disease diagnosis with accuracy.

Other physicians see a very different picture, and they have formed the International Lyme and Associated Disease Society (ILADS). These doctors, including me, have seen thousands of patients who had seemingly prolonged illnesses that were direct results of Lyme infection. This chronic version of the illness is much more difficult to treat than acute Lyme disease, often requiring multiple rounds of antibiotics for prolonged periods of time, sometimes intravenously. The unfortunate individuals who fall into this category of having chronic Lyme disease have been weakened by their disease to such an extent that we see many of the deficiencies and imbalances discussed earlier in this book—adrenal, thyroid, magnesium, food allergy, dysbiosis, and direct toxicities—all of them caused by both treatments and the Lyme organisms themselves.

As the patient with chronic Lyme disease becomes more and more depleted by multiple imbalances, a biochemical domino effect occurs in which each imbalance predisposes the body to the next, further depleting the patient and creating a vicious spiral downward. Ultimately this becomes so complicated that treatment for this condition has become a unique medical field, and the practitioners who provide this treatment are described as "Lyme literate." Some patients are so depleted that we can't even begin to give them antibiotics until we have recognized these deficiencies and built up their strength to the point where they are able to tolerate the antibiotics and respond properly. Many of these patients have negative tests for Lyme disease when they start treatment; however, these tests only measure the amount of antibodies the body has been able to create in order to counter the Lyme organism. Hence, if the immune system was weakened to the point that it could not produce these antibodies, the test would show no traces of them with our first measurements. Eventually, patients will test positive as their immune systems get stronger and treatment proceeds.

We have also come to realize that when the tick injects its secretions into us, it is not just Lyme bacteria that enter our bodies: it is extremely common for the parasite *Babesia,* the bacteria *Bartonella,* and other infective agents to be injected into us at the same time! We must be aware of these co-infections so that they can be diagnosed and treated along with the Lyme organisms. Also keep in mind that our new knowledge about biotoxicity, pioneered by Dr. Ritchie Shoemaker and discussed in Chapter 11, has allowed us to understand and treat this chronic illness with a deeper understanding of its complex biochemistry. Listed below are some of the most common symptoms of chronic Lyme disease.

### Common Symptoms of Chronic Lyme Disease

- Erythema chronicum migrans ( the "bull's-eye" rash present in only 30 percent of cases)
- Recurrent joint swelling and pain
- Cardiac conduction defects (atrioventricular blocks or arrhythmias)
- Neurological symptoms, including:
    Optic neuritis and atrophy
    Cranial neuritis (Bell's Palsy, affecting the 7th cranial nerve)
- Aseptic meningitis
- Radiculopathies (nerve root compression, especially at the cervical 5th and thoracic 8th–12th vertebral levels
- Cranial nerves 2, 3, and 6 effects
- Conjunctivitis, iritis, and uveitis (eye inflammations)
- Depression
- Memory loss
- Excessive daytime sleep
- Fatigue
- Extreme irritability and emotional lability (mood swings)
- Word-finding difficulties
- Spatial disorientation
- Photo- and phonophobia (sensitivity to light and sound)

With so many different symptoms possibly being presented, you can begin to see the problem inherent in making a diagnosis of Lyme disease. In the various states in which I have practiced, the majority of infectious disease specialists believe that Lyme disease is an uncommon event, so they are not inclined to diagnose or treat it. Worse, as they are the specialists in this area, this opinion has trickled down to most of the rank-and-file physicians so that they don't diagnose or treat it either. The Department of Health in every state, however, publishes a newsletter (called the *Morbidy and Mortality Report*) documenting the existence of hundreds of reported cases of Lyme disease. Since Lyme disease does not require mandatory reporting by physicians in most of those states, many Lyme experts believe that we really have ten to twenty times that amount of Lyme disease, most of which is going undiagnosed. This represents a considerable discrepancy in opinion, and a very serious problem as patients with a treatable disease are suffering for years with no diagnosis and no hope. To make the situation worse, and as with our toxic mold patients, when these unfortunate souls receive conventional medical care, they are usually told their problem is psychological and given antidepressants, which rarely work.

## MARK'S STORY

Mark, a cattle rancher, first came to see me many years ago when he was forty-eight. His main concerns were diminishing energy levels, which had been bothering him for several years. He also noted the new onset of severe headaches, nausea, chest pain, and abdominal pain. He had recently been hospitalized for two weeks, and thorough testing provided no clear diagnosis other than sleep apnea. His DHEA level when we started was only at 233 ng/dL (normal for his age would be closer to 650 ng/dL). He also showed a high mercury level of 15 mcg/g creatinine on the DMPS challenge test. He had only a moderate magnesium deficiency and mild hypoglycemia. Testing for food allergy and stool analysis did not provide any useful or additional information.

Despite treating all of these components, I could only help Mark become marginally better and he continued to wrestle with headaches, chest pain, and extreme fatigue. Symptoms fluctuated: Some days he could work a full day on his ranch, and other days he could barely function. He eventually went to the Mayo Clinic, where an exhaustive analysis showed no clear cause for his symptoms.

A visual contrast test showed the likelihood of biotoxicity, so I began treatment with cholestyramine and searched for causes of his biotoxicity. Despite a negative screening test for Lyme disease and a borderline Western blot test (the only accurate test for Lyme disease), I felt that chronic Lyme disease provided the best explanation for all of his symptoms. Mark agreed to treatment with a series of antibiotics. When we added Dr. Patricia Kane's detoxification program, consisting of intravenous treatments of phosphatidylcholine and glutathione, he began to improve much more rapidly. He also had several excellent responses to Christian religious healing services, but these responses did not last. Over a period of several years, our slow, continued work on detoxification—provided by a variety of health practitioners—led to even more consistent improvement. While I cannot say with absolute certainty that Mark has been wrestling with a chronic Lyme infection, his response to treatment for that condition, along with his symptoms, which would be difficult to explain in any other way, lead me to believe that this is indeed his diagnosis, and he agrees.

---

I present Mark's case as an example of the complexity in making some of these diagnoses, but also as an example of how a hopeful, persistent approach may lead to excellent results. As of this writing, Mark is able to work long, hard hours on his cattle ranch without headaches, chest pains, or fatigue, and he now has his life back.

I fear that thousands of unfortunate patients have been suffering with the symptoms of chronic Lyme disease without realizing it. The ILADS group has noted that the classic rash of Lyme disease may be present only one-third of the time, and that the standard tests are highly inaccurate. To underscore this, in the standard practice of medicine, when a Lyme test is requested by a physician, most labs only run a screening test for Lyme disease, which is incapable of recognizing the majority of patients who have the disease. By doing this screening, which is often negative, they do not go further to conduct the more accurate Western blot test. And even this test can be negative in many people with chronic Lyme disease. What a mess!

Much of the unwillingness to admit that we have a serious problem of chronic Lyme disease is underscored by an intense push by the insurance industry. These companies are loathe to pay for the expensive and prolonged intravenous treatments that may be necessary for a cure.

There is certainly more to say about chronic Lyme infection, but this is a start, and I refer you to other sources for further details at the end of this chapter. Remember, when you, or someone you love has been ill with symptoms that are so unusual that they seem to make no sense, one should always consider the possibility of Lyme disease with its attendant co-infections.

## NEW CONCEPTS THAT HELP US TO TREAT BACTERIAL INFECTIONS MORE EFFECTIVELY (OR REASONS WHY ANTIBIOTIC TREATMENTS MAY NOT WORK EFFECTIVELY)

Turning now to other forms of bacterial infections, I would first like to bring forth several newer medical concepts that may explain why so much controversy surrounds our understanding of these infections.

### Biofilm

The routine practice of microbiology consists of growing bacteria obtained from patients' bodies (in blood, urine, stool or skin) in the laboratory and then testing that growth with specific antibiotics to discover which ones would work best in each patient's case. We call that test, in standard medical practice, the culture and sensitivity report. This nice but simplistic system postulates that each infection is caused by a single type of bacteria that we can isolate and treat with precision. If only it was that easy.

Unfortunately, emerging evidence shows us that bacterial populations are actually mixed communities of different types of bacteria, sometimes including fungi, embedded in a matrix that it secretes around itself. We call this matrix a biofilm. We are learning that these complex biofilms are capable of protecting the bacteria from the various components of our immune system. To adequately treat them requires information we do not yet have: We have to be able to discern the makeup of these colonies, which requires diagnostic tools that are not yet available to most practicing clinicians. The good news is that many of these tools are under development and a brief catalogue of their names sounds like a sci-fi movie: denaturing gradient gel electrophoresis and high-performance liquid chromatography, polymerase chain reaction (PCR) and pyrosequencing, along with fluorescent in-situ-hybridization. The Fry Laboratories (www.frylabs.com) are now offering the first of these tests, and we are hopeful that this signals the emergence of many more.

In addition to accessing the most precise diagnostic tools, we will also need to understand the chemistry of the biofilm gel itself so we can keep it from blocking our treatments. Perhaps most important is our new awareness that 99 percent of the bacteria in nature (in our bodies) exist in the form of biofilm colonies, and only 1 percent are free-floating bacteria susceptible to our antibiotics. We will need to factor that knowledge into our treatment programs as we move into the future.

Understanding that difficult-to-eradicate microbes create, and hide, inside of thick biofilms gives us a new field to explore: by learning how to dissolve, or work with biofilm colonies, we are hopeful that we will create much more effective antibiotic treatment programs for Lyme disease and the co-infections.

## PANDAS

Another important set of bacterial infections that can contribute to chronic illness are the pediatric autoimmune and neurological diseases (PANDAS) caused by strep infections. In the past ten years, we have identified this condition in which a seemingly simple case of strep throat sets off a sudden change in behavior. This was first recognized in children but is being seen more often in adults as we have become more aware of its existence. In children, we find eating disorders, depression, anxiety, and bipolar behaviors suddenly appearing. We are also finding evidence of recent, unresolved strep infections (diagnosable with an ASO titer, a commonly available blood test, and with several more exotic tests as well). These children may respond dramatically to adequate doses of antibiotics provided over a longer-than-usual course of time. Children infected with PANDAS may also require intravenous immunoglobulin. Eventually, they may require a tonsillectomy for treatment, as the strep bacteria may lay dormant, or hide in the deep crypts of an infected tonsil.

## Cell-Wall-Deficient Bacteria

A third important "new" medical concept is that of *cell-wall-deficient bacteria*. The research demonstrating the reality of this phenomenon began in the late 1940s but never became popular, as it challenged the simplicity of the system already in place. Basically, we have learned over the years that many bacteria are capable of changing their shape and taking on the appearance of other forms as a part of their lifecycle. This means that they may look like common bacteria in one form, but appear fungal-like in others. They can also form microscopic cysts, which for all practical purposes hide them from our immune surveillance. Going back to Lyme disease, *Borrelia* is an example of a spirochete that can change into a cell-wall-deficient form. Yet another difficulty in successfully eradicating Lyme disease is that these bacteria are capable of morphing into a microscopic cystic phase, making it much more difficult to reach or eliminate them with simple, short courses of antibiotics, or by continuing to use antibiotics which had previously been effective for one specific form.

Several excellent textbooks have been written covering the idea of cell-wall-deficient bacteria. One of the more notable books is *Cell Wall Deficient Forms: Stealth Pathogens (1993)*, written by noted clinical microbiologist Lida Mattman. Another slightly older text is *Cell Wall-Deficient Bacteria* (1982), by Gerald Domingue. Despite the publishing of these well-documented textbooks, most microbiologists and clinicians have been slow to embrace this field of study. But we can't wait much longer. This concept may help us to better understand what we are facing in illness. We will discuss these cell-wall-deficient bacteria in more detail in Chapter 21, when we talk about cancers and the pioneering research by Dr. Virginia Livingston.

## VIRAL INFECTIONS

Bacteria are single-celled organisms with a nucleus and a cell membrane. They, like all cells, have to metabolize, make new structures, obtain nutrients, remove wastes, and "breathe" in one form or another. Viruses, on the other hand, are a different critter entirely. They consist of a core of genetic material, either RNA or DNA, so that the virus can replicate itself, and each virus is wrapped in a coat of protein. A virus doesn't have a nucleus, really, nor does it need to "breathe" or carry out other typical functions of cells. In fact, it isn't clear if a virus is really alive or not.

Once again, it is our intact immune system that allows us to recognize the foreign nature of the virus and fight it off. Usually it does so relatively easily, and the majority of viral infections, when they are eradicated, are gone. We may even develop long-lasting immunity to that virus. However, there is a whole family of viruses that are uniquely difficult for us to deal with. They are the herpes viruses, and we number them from 1 to 8, each with a different name and slightly different focus of infection. The table "Herpes Family of Viruses" illustrates these herpes virus types and their common traits.

| HERPES FAMILY OF VIRUSES | | |
|---|---|---|
| **HERPES VIRUS SPECIES** | **COMMON ABBREVIATION** | **DISEASES CAUSED BY THE VIRUS** |
| Herpes simplex virus-1 | HSV-1 | Oral herpes |
| Herpes simplex virus-2 | HSV-2 | Genital herpes |
| Varicella-Zoster virus | VZV | Chicken pox, shingles |
| Epstein-Barr virus | EBV | Mononucleosis |
| Cytomegalovirus | CMV | "monolike" flu |
| Human herpes virus-6 | HHV-6 | roseola, multiple sclerosis (MS), fatigue |
| Human herpes virus-7 | HHV-7 | Pityriasis rosea |
| Human herpes virus-8 | HHV-8 | Kaposi's sarcoma |

Most of us are familiar with many of these viral strains. What the members of this family have in common is the ability to *hide* from our immune system so that we don't completely recognize or eradicate them. In fact, new research shows us that these viruses actually have methods for altering the structure of their DNA to facilitate this hiding process. What we have known for quite some time is that when the virus feels threatened by our immune system, it can move deep into our nerve cells and wait until the immune surveillance goes away. The most obvious example of this is shingles, in which the virus goes directly into the nerve ganglions and specifically infects nerve tissue. Sometimes the virus lingers, causing a rather severe pain called *postherpetic neuralgia.*

Years ago, when chronic fatigue syndrome first began to appear, it was proposed that chronic Epstein-Barr virus (EBV) was a cause. By 1982 Dr. Jay Goldstein, who pioneered some of the early understanding and treatment of chronic fatigue, provided evidence for this connection. Unfortunately, EBV is a common infection, and conventional medicine dismissed it as an irrelevant cause of chronic illness since "everyone" had it. It was also true at that time that we physicians had little to nothing to offer in the way of treatment, so this component of chronic fatigue lay neglected.

Several recent developments have spurred our interest in chronic viral infections as a component of chronic illness. One is new research by Dr. Jose Montoya, an infectious disease specialist from Stanford University. He administered large doses of antiviral antibiotics (Valcyte and Valtrex) to chronic fatigue patients for six months, and patients with chronic fatigue syndrome that had tested positive for human herpes virus 6 (HHV-6) and EBV initially showed significant improvement. Unfortunately, those benefits did not hold, but the research gives us hope that successful treatments may be just around the corner. While it is true that most people test positive for exposure to these viruses, those with chronic fatigue have significantly higher viral titers on blood tests, and newer methods of detection for these viruses are more accurate. Our detection methods are still nowhere near as accurate as we need them to be, but they are getting better.

Recently, a unique treatment for some of these viruses was developed by Dr. Joe Brewer, an infectious disease specialist in Kansas City. Brewer created a specific chemical compound called a *transfer factor* for each virus he wanted to treat: HHV-6; CMV; EBV; and herpes viruses 1, 2, and 3. Transfer factors are also called *immunomodulators*. They are chemicals that are taken from animals or humans that are naturally immune to or have developed immunity against certain diseases. Cows, for example, do not get the viral infections that we have been discussing and that Dr. Brewer was targeting for treatment. He injected a purified form of each of these viruses into pregnant cows' udders, so that they made antibodies to the virus. He then withdrew the antibodies from the cows' udders and purified them into a form called a *transfer factor,* which is now available for oral use from several different companies. Dr. Brewer discovered that if patients took the transfer factor for these viruses for six months, some of them got well but soon relapsed. If they took it for a year, 40 percent were cured. After eighteen months of taking transfer factor, 60 percent were cured. The longer the product was used, the less the chance of relapse. For the first time, true cures of these chronic viral illnesses were possible. Even though a complete cure takes longer, those who respond usually note marked improvement after four months.

## KENDRA'S STORY

Thiry-five-year-old Kendra came to my office with a history of sporadic fatigue and cognitive difficulties, along with episodes of asthma. She had already been treated previously for mercury toxicity and had responded well to chelation treatments. Her DHEA level was low at 192 ng/dL (normal for her age should have been around 650 ng/dL), so I provided DHEA supplementation, and I also treated her food allergies. These measures led to modest benefits, until we discovered an elevated EBV viral titer (a blood test showing antibodies to EBV virus and quantifying it) and began her on transfer factor therapy specific for EBV virus.

When Kendra began taking the transfer factor, she became much more fatigued and had a recurrence of most of her symptoms. While this is of concern, it is not unusual and actually confirms EBV as a significant component of her illness. If it wasn't, she would have had no reaction to the transfer factor at all. By themselves, if there has been no viral exposure, transfer factors cause no side effects at all. If a patient experiences viral-type symptoms when she begins taking them, this can only mean that she does indeed have that virus in her system, and her system is now being stimulated to fight it. The symptoms however, if intense, represent an overstimulation, and this is why we sometimes have to cut down on the dosage until that immune system becomes more comfortable and tolerable. So we decreased the starting dose, and she cut back on the frequency of taking it to every third day until she was able to tolerate the transfer factor with no negative effects. Slowly but steadily, over several months, she was able to work up to the full dose of supplement, and by the fourth month reported marked improvement in all of her symptoms. At that point, she discovered that if she missed a few doses, her symptoms would return, only to disappear when she took the dose more faithfully. Kendra was able to discontinue the transfer factor therapy after eighteen months and her progress held steady.

## GcMAF: AN INNOVATIVE APPROACH
## TO IMPROVING IMMUNE SYSTEM FUNCTIONS

A new and exciting breakthrough in treating chronic fatigue syndrome (also called myalgic encephalomyelitis or ME) is through understanding another way in which viruses may "disable" a part of the immune system from functioning properly.

GcMAF stands for GcProtein macrophage activating factor. GcProtein is also called *vitamin D binding protein* (VDBP), and it is the important precursor for macrophage activating factor (in other words, vitamin D if functioning normally, stimulates microphages to do their job properly). Macrophages are one of the most important lines of white blood cells that are critical in our recognition of foreign invaders and our ability to destroy them and thus crucial to supporting our immune and disease-fighting systems. It turns out that viruses (and some bacteria and tumor cells) can make a unique enzyme called *alpha-N-acetylgalac-tosaminidase*, which has been given the less intimidating nickname of "nagalase." This enzyme prevents GcProtein from being converted into GcMAF and this leads to immunosuppression—the immune system is unable to create the macrophages they so desperately need to eradicate viruses. The induction of increased nagalase activity by viruses and some bacteria may well be the central adaptive mechanism that "blinds" the immune system to the presence of these pathogens. The good news is that we can measure nagalase activity with a simple blood test.

We have recently gained access to the use of GcMAF in patients who have high levels of nagalase activity. We have found that many of them who have been ill for years with chronic viral and bacterial infections, many of whom have been diagnosed with chronic fatigue syndrome, respond well to the administration of GcMAF with significant clinical improvement, giving hope to many chronic fatigue sufferers that their long-standing immune suppression may be relieved.

## MYCOBACTERIA AND CHLAMYDIA PNEUMONIAE

*Mycobacteria* and *Chlamydia pneumoniae* are very small infectious organisms—between the size of a viral particle and a bacterium. The most common illness caused by these organisms is walking pneumonia, also called *atypical pneumonia.*

We have also recognized that Gulf War illness, another severe, chronic illness largely ignored or denied by the medical profession, is strongly associated with some unusual mycobacterial infections. This connection was discovered in work pioneered by Garth Nicholson, the president and chief scientific officer at the Institute of Molecular Medicine in South Laguna Beach, California. We have learned over time that many of our Gulf War returnees need to be treated with an average of six rounds of antibiotics, lasting six weeks each, to achieve a complete cure. Many chronic illnesses have been linked to these infections, including amyotrophic lateral sclerosis (ALS, or Lou Gehrig's disease), autoimmune illnesses, such as rheumatoid arthritis, lupus, and scleroderma, and chronic fatigue. Multiple sclerosis has been specifically linked to persistent *Chlamydia pneumoniae* infections, and successfully treated with the use of antibiotics in many cases. These infections can be diagnosed, again, with a simple blood test available from most laboratories. What is new is that we are learning that we may need to treat these infections aggressively in order to help those who have been incapacitated for many years with undiagnosed conditions.

## HALLIE'S STORY

Hallie first came to my office five years ago, when she was twenty-eight years old. She had been diagnosed by a rheumatologist as having fibromyalgia and was told she should just grow up and live with it. Her symptoms began six years before, when she was involved in a motor vehicle accident and sustained injuries to her neck and upper shoulder. As time went on, she got worse and the joint pain increased and spread to other areas. It is not unusual for an injury to progress to full-blown fibromyalgia, as it did for Hallie.

I began treating her with osteopathic manipulation (see Chapter 17) for her neck and shoulder areas, and discovered a low DHEA level of 110 ng/dL (for her age, it should have been about 800 ng/dL). I also noted a low magnesium level of 31.2 mEq/L (the normal range is 33.9 to41.0 mEq/L). We supplemented her with DHEA at a dose of 50 mg each morning and provided magnesium taurate in 125 mg capsules, two at bedtime. After several months of treatment, she was somewhat better, but we were still trying to achieve complete healing. As I described earlier, when really young people get chronic fatigue and fibromyalgia, most of them turn out to have had an EBV infection, even if they were unaware of having mononucleosis as a teenager. So we then measured her Epstein-Barr viral levels and the lab reported them to be extremely high. I prescribed transfer factors for her, and within several months she returned to our office describing marked improvement in all areas. She continued her transfer factors for several years, telling us she was "almost" well. We continued our diagnostic exploration, and after making the additional diagnoses of a chronic Candida infection and low cortisol, both of which were treated, she completed the final stages of her healing journey, with complete relief from her symptoms of fibromyalgia and chronic fatigue. At that time I was not yet aware of the possible benefits of frequency specific microcurrent (FSM) in fibromyalgia that occurred following neck injury, which we will discuss in Chapter 18.

Of our various interventions, Hallie considered taking the transfer factors for her EBV infection as providing the most impressive results. She had no memory of having had mononucleosis as a teenager, and this is not unusual in our practice. This case emphasizes that when a youngster comes to me with a history of not feeling well since high school, this is often a tip-off that we need to look for residual, chronic EBV infection and treat it. The good news is that now we can. The other infection often missed in youngsters who are languishing for no clear reason is Lyme disease with its co-infections.

Once again, as we explore these concepts, we have hope. When a teenager or young adult presents to me with chronic fatigue and fibromyalgia, an increasingly common occurrence in my practice unfortunately, usually we find EBV infection, even if she was never formally diagnosed with mononucleosis. By the time I see the patient, several years may have elapsed, and as her body has weakened, we find depleted adrenal and thyroid function. By treating these three areas—the EBV infection and the adrenal and thyroid hormone imbalances—many patients recover completely within just a few months. It is inspiring to see youngsters who have had their lives so limited by illness resume their lives wholeheartedly.

## FURTHER READING

Brewer, Joseph, Administration of Transfer Factor for Human Herpes Virus-6 (HHV-6) in patients with Chronic Fatigue Syndrome and HHV6 Viremia, www.immunitytoday.com.hhv6article.html.

Goldstein, Jay A. *Betrayal by the Brain: The Neurologic Basis of Chronic Fatigue Syndrome, Fibromyalgia Syndrome and Related Neural Network Disorders.* New York: Routledge, 1996.

Makris, Katina I., *Out of the Woods: Healing Lyme Disease—Body, Mind & Spirit,* Elite Books, Santa Rosa, CA, 2011.

Montoya, Jose, *Use of Valganciclovir in Patients with Elevated Antibody Titers against Human Herpes 6 (HHV-6) And Epstein-Barr Virus (EBV)* A randomized, placebo-controlled, double blind study at Stanford University, www.vicd.info/clinicaltrial.html, 2007.

LymeDisease.org publishes a quarterly journal called the *Lyme Times* at www.lymedisease.org; ILADS can be accessed through www.ilads.org.

For a more in-depth discussion of Lyme disease, please visit the website for the Mendocino Coast District Hospital; I presented a two-hour discussion on Lyme disease for the hospital, which was filmed by public television; go to www.mcdh.org and click on Health & Wellness, then go to Video on Demand for this free presentation.

For transfer factor information and availability visit www.researched nutritionals.com.

# CHAPTER 13

# Amino Acids and Neurotransmitter Imbalances

## This Is Getting on My Nerves

The word *neurotransmitter* refers to those natural chemicals that assist in the transmission of electrical impulses through our nerves (neurons). When the electrical impulse that fires through every nerve in our body reaches the outer cellular limit of a neuron, or nerve cell, the energy of that impulse is translated into a chemical reaction. The chemicals involved in these reactions are our neurotransmitters. These neurotransmitters then cross the microscopic gap between nerves—called a synapse. When the chemical reaches the other side of the synapse, it again is translated into a fired-up electrical impulse, and the communication process continues. Dozens of neurotransmitter chemicals are known, but several are considered of overriding importance to our health.

The best known of these neurotransmitters is probably *serotonin*, which plays a central role in preventing depression, controlling pain, and allowing sleep. Almost everyone is familiar with the antidepressant medications widely advertised on television: Zoloft, Prozac, Paxil, Effexor, Celexa, Lexapro, and Cymbalta. All of these belong to the family of antidepressants called *selective serotonin reuptake inhibitors* (SSRIs). While the full name is a mouthful, it accurately reflects what these medications do. When the chemical, in this case serotonin, reaches its destination at the end of the synapse, it has completed its job. The serotonin is then normally broken down by enzymes so that more serotonin can be released from the other end of the neuron, and the process can continue.

If we slow down or inhibit this enzymatic process by using SSRIs, we artificially increase the amount of serotonin available in the synapse, and the brain gets the impression that it has all of the serotonin it needs. As the name suggests, the reuptake of serotonin is thus inhibited. What most physicians seem to ignore is that this artificially created sense that we have an adequate level of serotonin will eventually send a message to the brain that it is doing fine, and that we don't have to keep making more. So the chemical process by which serotonin is made basically takes a vacation, and what we see, clinically, is that people on these medications need to take more and more of their medication to get the same effect; or they must switch medications, where eventually this same process is repeated. Wouldn't it make more sense to give the body the raw materials by which it could manufacture more of what it needs? Yes, it would, and this is actually possible.

Several physicians, including Marty Hinz and Tom Uncini at Neuro-Research in Duluth, Minnesota, have been studying this problem for the last twenty years. While their focus has been primarily on obesity, which they see as a major neurotransmitter deficiency disease, they have also observed that a wide variety of medical problems, including fibromyalgia, chronic fatigue, depression, anxiety, anorexia, bulimia, panic attacks, migraine headaches, Parkinson's disease, PMS, obsessive-compulsive disorder, IBS, and Crohn's disease, also seem to have neurotransmitter deficiency as an important feature.

Using a computer model with hundreds of thousands of clinical results, Hinz and Uncini have put together combinations of amino acids in specific proportions, each designed to stimulate the body to improve its production of the key neurotransmitters. The focus of their research is not only on serotonin, which we've been discussing, but also on dopamine, which in turn is made into epinephrine and norepinephrine. These four neurotransmitters, which they call the master neurotransmitters, are the focus of their innovative treatment program.

I have included diagrams of the basic chemistry of the synthesis of these neurotransmitters in Figures 13.1 and 13.2. What I hope you can see at a glance is that the process of converting these amino acids into our key neurotransmitters is a relatively simple one, involving only or two steps in each case. That is the main idea I would like to convey in these diagrams. For those who wish to look at this chemistry in more detail, you can see in Figure 13.1 that the amino acid tryptophan is converted into 5-hydroxy-tryptophan (5-HTP), which in turn is converted into serotonin. Figure 13.2 shows the equally straightforward process of converting the amino acid tyrosine into Dopa, which in turn is converted into dopamine and then into norepinephrine and then into epinephrine. I hope you can see that these chemical conversions are actually fairly straightforward.

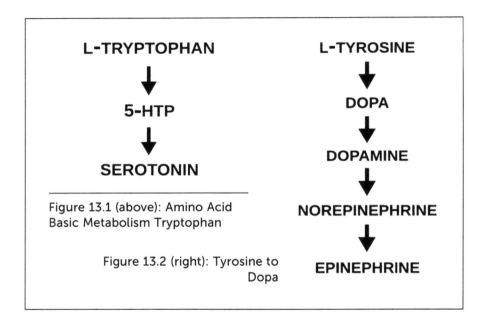

Figure 13.1 (above): Amino Acid Basic Metabolism Tryptophan

Figure 13.2 (right): Tyrosine to Dopa

Hinz and Uncini have discovered that by providing patients 5-HTP and tyrosine, which are precursors for neurotransmitters (in other words, they are necessary for their synthesis and directly converted into them) in carefully orchestrated patient-specific doses, the body can make what it needs. These materials are provided as oral supplements, and by adding the amino acid cysteine and several cofactors that nourish these reactions also as oral supplements, they can indeed get the body to make more of the required neurotransmitters. They report remarkable success in treating all of the conditions noted above, and I can confirm from my own experience that this is an effective treatment for many chronically ill patients.

## KATY'S STORY

Katy first came to see me in 1997, when she was forty-one years old. A year and a half prior, she had been diagnosed by an ENT specialist (ear, nose, and throat doctor) as having temporal mandibular joint dysfunction (TMJ) and had recently been referred to an oral surgeon. TMJ is the common designation for jaw pain accompanied by clicking and popping in the jaw joints, a sense that the teeth are not properly aligned when the jaw closes, and an inability to open the jaw adequately or chew down on hard foods. Uncertain that surgery was necessary, Katy was referred to me by a colleague for osteopathic cranial manipulation. She began to respond immediately to treatment, and within a few months could chew apples again; within four months she was essentially well. She noted that for the first time in years her jaw no longer popped. Although this part of the story is a digression on my part, and probably not related to what happened next, it does present an opportunity to give another example of the potential benefits of cranial manipulation, which we discuss in Chapter 17. I continued to follow Katy and she has never required the skills of an oral surgeon.

Several years later, however, Katy came to me with acute hip and knee pain, which slowly progressed into pains over much of her body. Within a year, in April 2000, this condition was formally diagnosed as fibromyalgia. It was one of the worst cases of fibromyalgia I've ever seen, a diagnosis and degree of severity confirmed by several rheumatologists. She was unable to continue working at her job. She is one of the few patients for whom I had to provide large doses of pain medication and muscle relaxants for years, until she finally improved. It was a very long and arduous journey. Her muscles went into spasms so intense that they were palpably rock-hard and these episodes lasted for days at a time. Extensive osteopathic treatments could only relieve the pain and spasms for short periods of time. Our usual evaluation and treatment, all documented with laboratory testing, helped only briefly. I looked at and treated her adrenal and thyroid deficiencies (thyroiditis confirmed), mercury toxicity, mycoplasma infection, perimenopausal hormonal deficiencies, EBV infection, Candida and bacterial pathogens, and fatty acid imbalances. None of the treatments for these deficiencies did much to bring Katy out of her compromised state. Other treatments such as the use of colostrum, penicillamine, cholestyramine, and low-dose Naltrexone also had no effect. Her weight fluctuated wildly with fifty-pound swings that were baffling to both of us.

A year after her symptoms began, Katy also developed unusual paresthesias, which are sensations of numbness and tingling, over her facial areas and extremities. Neurologists had no diagnosis to offer, but after quite a bit of experimenting I found that the medication Topamax would at least bring these symptoms under control. Consultations at Mayo Clinic and elsewhere were confusing, contradictory, and generally unhelpful. Her gallbladder, filled with small stones, was removed in 2003, with no additional benefits to her whole system.

Approximately six years into Katy's illness and still treading water, I began the amino acid protocol, providing her with 5-HTP and tyrosine so that her body could make more of the essential neurotransmitters. Within a month, she was 50 percent better, and then continued to improve significantly. Within a year of starting the amino acid treatments she was able to return to full-time employment in an executive position, and she has really enjoyed getting her life back. She is not completely well yet, but with the addition of the methylation protocol (which I will discuss in the next chapter), slowly and surely her symptoms are disappearing so that she is now 75 to 80 percent better. I have repeatedly commended Katy for hanging in there with me as we attempted to figure out which imbalances were contributing to her illness. And, as she pointed out to me, "What choice did I have?" This is an excellent example of how, as our knowledge expands, we are able to provide effective treatments today that didn't exist years ago, when Katy and I started on our journey. The profound improvement provided by the amino acid treatment protocol clearly initiated her return to health.

---

Hinz and Uncini have noted that the need for increased amounts of neurotransmitters comes from damage to the nerves themselves. They further note that neurotoxins, heavy metal toxicity, and even food reactions (all of which I have described as important to the understanding of chronic illness) deplete and compromise the ability of these nerves to function. The prolonged use of medications, especially antidepressants, amphetamines, migraine medications, ephedra, caffeine, nicotine, and alcohol, further compromises the body's ability to make and sustain neurotransmitter production.

While I agree with this portion of their hypothesis, Hinz and Uncini also state that once the amino acids have started working, they have to be taken for prolonged periods of time because the nerves have been permanently damaged. That has not been my observation. Nerves can, and do, heal. I have repeatedly noticed that when you add other protocols to the improvement in neurotransmitter function, including detoxification, hormonal rebalance, treatment of occult infections, general improvement of immune function, and restoration of overall hormonal balance, most patients can maintain their own state of health once it has been restored. They do not seem to need to use these amino acids for long stretches of time. The addition of the technologies of FSM and LENS, which I will discuss later in Chapter 18, add yet another opportunity to provide healing for inflamed and injured nerves.

I do find it useful to prescribe these amino acids to all patients who have been on antidepressants for prolonged periods of time and to consider their use in all chronic illness. The amino acids have also been uniquely helpful for patients with Parkinson's disease, where these same principles apply. As we have seen in depression, where the continuing use of antidepressants depletes the body's supply of neurotransmitters, we know, too, that prolonged use of medication for Parkinson's disease, which is standard medical therapy, is also associated with a gradual weakening effect of those medications over time. This means that treatment dosages need to be steadily increased and additional medications added to continue the benefits of therapy. The use of specific amino acid therapy for these patients has enabled us to lessen the amount of medication needed and to see improved effects of the medication already in use, over time.

## BERNICE'S STORY

I first saw Bernice when she was sixty-one years old. She had developed Parkinson's disease three years prior and had tried a variety of alternative treatments. These included the treatment of mercury toxicity and the regular use of intravenous glutathione, working up to doses of 2,500 mg given three times per week. Although she did fairly well with these treatments, her tremors and difficulty with walking and movement slowly worsened, and it became more and more difficult for her to function.

She was quite holistically inclined but eventually accepted a trial of conventional medication along with her alternative program. She was initially given the medication Requip, and later, following consultation with a neurologist, was switched to Sinemet 25/100, given three times daily. The improvement with conventional medication was dramatic: Bernice was able to move with considerable ease and found that her tremors had decreased significantly. Over time, however, as is often the case, the benefits of medication did not hold, and higher and higher doses of medication were required to produce the same benefits.

Unfortunately, the side effects of the higher dosage of medication were becoming more difficult for Bernice to tolerate. So we began the amino acid protocol, using the supplements called D5 and Cysreplete in small doses. These materials simply consist of the amino acids tyrosine and 5-HTP in specific proportions, along with cysteine and several other vitamins and minerals. We start with tiny doses of each, and slowly increase the dose on a weekly schedule until we optimize our results. If we see improvement and feel that we can do even better, we can provide urine testing of the neurotransmitters to "tweak" our prescription of the amino acids; for about 20 percent of our patients, this is a helpful addition to the program. As these amino acids are natural supplements, we see very few side effects, even at high doses.

Within a few weeks on this protocol, Bernice was able to decrease her medication to her initial levels and was clinically even better, with virtually no tremors and a smooth walking gait. She told me that the amino acids definitely agreed with her. There was no doubt that the amino acids extended the benefits of her Parkinson medication appreciably. Over the last three years, these benefits have continued unabated, and Bernice remains delighted with her improvement on less medication.

---

As you can see, the depletion of neurotransmitters is a common component of many chronic illnesses, and by understanding and using the appropriate amino acids, we can greatly improve this aspect of health care for our patients.

## FURTHER READING

Braverman, Eric. *The Edge Effect: Achieve Total Health and Longevity with the Balanced Brain Advantage.* New York: Sterling, 2005.

Hinz, Marty, Stein, Alvin and Uncini, Thomas, Relative nutritional deficiencies associated with centrally active monoamines, *International Journal of General Medicine,* May, 2011, vol 2012:5 pp. 413–430.

Hinz, Marty, Stein Alvin, Neff, Robert, et al., Treatment of attention deficit hyperactivity disorder with monoamine amino acid precursors and organic cation transporter assay interpretation, *Neuropsychiatric Disease and Treatment,* Jan 2011, Vol 2011:7(1) pp 31–38.

Hinz, Marty, Stein, Alvin, and Uncini, Thomas, Amino acid management of Parkinson's disease: a case study, *International Journal of General Medicine,* Feb 2011, Vol 2011:4 pp 165–174.

For doctors, CHK Nutrition's website provides a host of neurotransmitter treatment materials. You can browse their products online at NeuroReplete.com or call them at (877) 626-2220.

# CHAPTER 14

# Methylation: A Key to Understanding Chronic Illness

## Got Methylation?

The term *methylation chemistry* is likely unfamiliar to you. However, when it comes to health, it is a subject of great importance. Understanding this process is essential for diagnosing imbalances in these essential chemical reactions and for discovering what we need to do to improve these reactions.

The word *methylation* simply refers to the process of adding a methyl "group" to another molecule. A methyl group is simply a chemical molecule composed of a carbon atom (C) surrounded by, or bound to, three hydrogen (H) atoms, with one free "bond" area left open. This is shown in the usual way that chemical formulas are written in Figure 14.1.

These four atoms act as a unit, and moving this unit around by adding it or subtracting it from other chemical molecules is what we define as *methylation*. The importance of this unit is that it is biochemically essential to some very important processes in the body: namely, detoxification, the creation of energy, quenching free radicals, and repairing and restoring damaged DNA. It turns

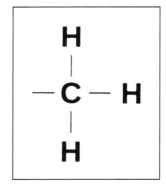

Figure 14.1: Methyl Group

out, actually, that hundreds of crucial chemical reactions in the body require the normal functioning of this methyl group give-and-take for us to be healthy.

For any specific methylation reaction (for example, melatonin, which is vital in allowing us to sleep properly, is created by methylating serotonin), we must use up some of these methyl groups. Once used up, obviously, we have to make more methyl groups because after we use that melatonin we will need to keep making more of it. Therefore, let us view this as a vital, ongoing process that requires a continuous supply of methyl groups, which we must create constantly for our chemistry to function properly. Since what follows consists of a fair degree of biochemical sophistication, you can skip ahead to less intimidating information if you'd like. On the other hand, if you can pluck up a little courage, I would like to try to walk you through this material. If you can understand even pieces of this information, it will allow this whole area to make a lot more sense to you, and you will better understand our therapeutic strategies and your options for treatment.

Let's plunge into this biochemistry and start with the amino acid methionine, to which the body adds another methyl group to create SAM (or SAMe, chemical shorthand for S-adenosyl methionine). SAM is a critically important methyl *donor,* or contributor, so that whenever the body needs methyl groups, it calls on that molecule (SAM) to provide them. Once SAM has given up its methyl group, it becomes SAH, which is short for S-adenosyl homocysteine, which in turn has to be

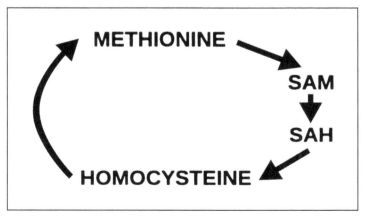

Figure 14.2: Basic Methylation Cycle to Create SAM

converted back into methionine by several more steps, so that this whole process can continue. Figure 14.2 illustrates this process.

Despite the long chemical names, the basic process here is simply a recycling of one molecule into another. As long as this cycle can continue functioning, unimpeded, life is good. But if the body cannot keep moving this cycle along properly, homocysteine or SAH may build up, and this creates a serious problem. We have known for many years now that an excess of homocysteine is inflammatory to the body and is associated with atherosclerosis (the buildup of plaque in our arteries) and other out-of-control inflammatory processes.

For this cycle to function properly, another cycle that interfaces with this one has to work in tandem. To convert or change homocysteine back into methionine, we need adequate amounts of an enzyme called *methionine synthase* (MS) and that enzyme requires adequate amounts of vitamin B12 and a derivative of folic acid, 5-CH3THF (short for

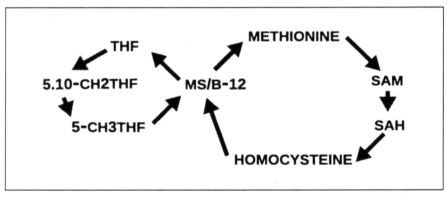

Figure 14.3: How the Folic Acid Cycle Interfaces with the Basic Methylation Cycle

5-methyl tetrahydrofolate) to do so. Combining these cycles as they interface looks like Figure 14.3.

Please hang tight; we're almost done with this chemistry lesson. Without focusing on the details of these cycles, you can see that they fit together like gears, and that each of these gears has to mesh properly with the others for the cycles to function properly.

The next crucial part of this chemistry is what the body *does* with

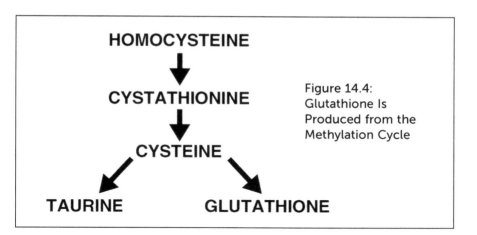

HOMOCYSTEINE

CYSTATHIONINE

Figure 14.4:
Glutathione Is
Produced from the
Methylation Cycle

CYSTEINE

TAURINE          GLUTATHIONE

homocysteine when it can't or doesn't remake methionine, which is depicted in Figure 14.4.

Depending on its needs, the body makes either glutathione or taurine. Glutathione is a critical material for the body and is central for detoxification and a host of other essential chemical reactions that cannot occur without it. Taurine, on the other hand, moves these reactions into another sphere, called the *transulfuration pathway,* and hence we lose the opportunity to make more glutathione, which is so important for us.

Believe it or not, what I have presented thus far is a gross simplification of this process. The point of going into this detail is to share my excitement about some newly learned information that allows us to identify exactly where these chemical reactions are blocked up, or stuck, and use this information to provide us with natural treatments that can keep the body methylating properly, allowing hundreds of vital biochemical reactions to be maximally optimized.

Hopefully, now you can understand the basic concept of methylation and some of the simple chemistry that underlies it. With this understanding, let us review the historical background that led us to this area of study.

Although we have long known that methylation is a vital biochemical process, affecting every cell in the body, its key importance in understanding many chronic medical conditions is a rather new discovery. Working with what are called *neurodegenerative diseases,* such as Parkinson's disease, Alzheimer's dementia, and multiple sclerosis, in the late 1990s Dr. Amy Yasko from Bethel, Maine, began to make some breakthroughs with her superb understanding of methylation chemistry. When presented with the opportunity to treat an autistic child, Amy applied her technology and understanding with surprising results, and this led to many years of success with helping autistic children to heal. She discovered that the majority of these children had genetic and biochemical "blocks" that prevented them from making the glutathione they needed, and that by providing them with the raw materials that their bodies required, most of them improved significantly. She speculated that other conditions, including fibromyalgia and chronic fatigue, might be connected to this inability to methylate properly.

In 2003, an engineer named Rich Van Konynenburg picked up on this idea and showed that if you analyzed all of the known biochemical disruptions of fibromyalgia and chronic fatigue syndrome, virtually every component could be explained by difficulties with methylation chemistry. He suggested that "blockage" of parts of the methylation pathway would prevent the body from making glutathione (which it requires for energy) properly and that by using some of the same natural materials that Dr. Yasko was using for autistic children, perhaps they could recover their health.

I first heard Rich present this hypothesis at a medical meeting in August 2007, and I was so intrigued with the logic and simplicity of his ideas that when I got home from the meeting, I immediately placed fifty-one patients with fibromyalgia and chronic fatigue syndrome on the five supplements that Rich extracted from Amy Yasko's work and described as a "simplified methylation protocol." Essentially, these five materials consist of several forms of vitamin B12 and several forms of folic acid (another vitamin in the B family). After several months of taking these supplements, 70 percent of my patients had improved, and of those who improved, 20 percent were *much* better. These results were so obviously important that we proposed a research project (which was graciously funded by the Ratna Ling Study Group) to study the science of methylation in these patients and learn more about what we were doing.

Since the original fifty-one patients had already received these supplements, I offered these supplements to thirty new patients, all of whom had fibromyalgia and chronic fatigue. All of these patients had had some success with the treatment program described in this book, with 30 to 60 percent improvement of their symptoms. While delighted with this improvement, all of them were still hopeful that they could do even better with additional treatments. So all of them had gotten better and were understandably not yet satisfied with what we had achieved. We were going to look at their methylation chemistry and genetics before we started, and then have them take these methylation supplements for six months. During this time, we would remeasure their methylation chemistry results at three months and then six months, and compare their progress with their chemistry laboratory testing. I was privileged to have been able to present this research at the annual scientific meeting for the American Academy of Environmental Medicine in October 2009.

First of all, not a single patient had normal methylation chemistry to start with, and all had abnormal methylation genetics, which was measured in Dr. Yasko's laboratory.

When we looked at their initial laboratory work, done by the Health Diagnostics and Research Institute in Amboy, New Jersey, the majority started with a low glutathione level (twenty-five out of thirty patients, or 83 percent, were low). The actual levels, which normally range from 3.8 to 5.5 micromol/L averaged 3.2 micromol/L in our patients. After three months, twenty-nine out of thirty patients had improved their glutathione levels (97 percent) to an average of 3.8 micromol/L.

SAM, which I have explained is of critical importance in methylation as the main methyl donor, was low initially in twenty out of thirty patients, and improved in twenty-seven of our thirty patients, which represents an increase of 90 percent in just three months! (See Figure 14.6 on page 169.)

By the end of six months, these numbers had continued to improve, significantly. By this time, the glutathione had risen to an average of 4.3 micromol/L (remember, their starting average was 3.2, so this was an improvement of 34 percent in that crucial metabolite). The SAM had risen to an average of 238 micromol/dL (from a starting level of 217 micromol/dL—an improvement of 10 percent). To put this in a different perspective, when we started, twenty-five of our thirty patients

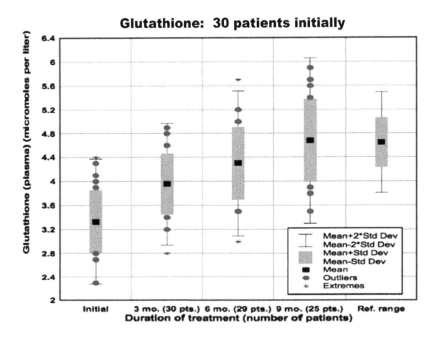

Figure 14.5. Improvement in Glutathione Levels with Methylation Protocol

were low in glutathione, and twenty out of thirty were low in SAM. At the completion of six months, only five patients were low in glutathione, only one patient failed to improve their glutathione level, and only four were low in SAM. The other methylation chemistry measures, including folic acid and folinic acid, all improved dramatically.

This is all well and good, but did these patients *feel* any better? At the start of our project, we asked all of our patients to rate, on a scale of 1 to 10, five main areas: their energy, sleep, mental clarity, pain, and overall sense of well-being. (See Figures 14.6 through 14.9.)

After three months, they rated these areas again, and the figures showed improvement in energy in 77 percent of patients, improvement in sleep in 65 percent, improvement in mental clarity in 73 percent, decrease in pain in 54 percent, and an overall sense of improvement in 70 percent. These gains held up nicely at the six-month evaluation.

From a different perspective, 83 percent told us they were improved (meaning 15 to 50 percent better), and of those who improved, 27 per-

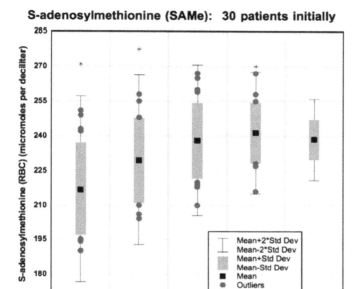

Figure 14.6

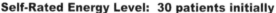

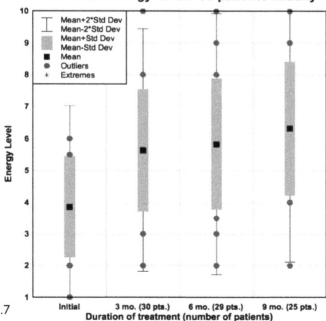

Figure 14.7

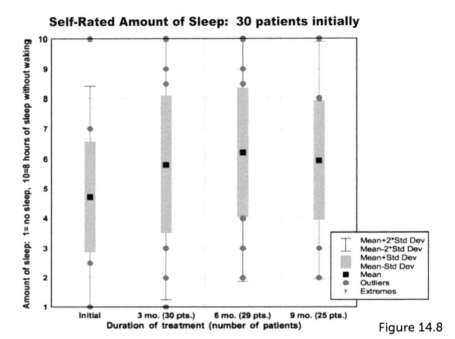

Figure 14.8

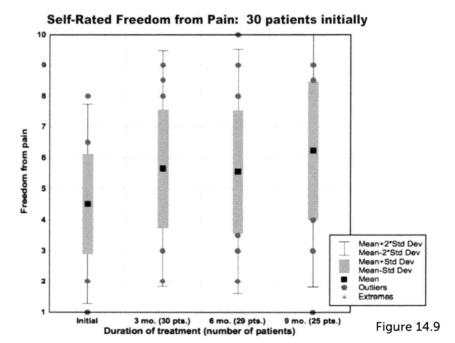

Figure 14.9

cent were *really* improved (meaning 50 to 100 percent better). The *average* improvement, at six months, was found to be 48 percent.

This is the basic question that we were attempting to answer: *Is the presence of abnormal methylation chemistry important to the development of fibromyalgia and chronic fatigue syndrome?* This has been answered with clarity: Yes. Clearly, abnormalities in methylation chemistry are common, almost universal, in our patients with chronic fatigue and fibromyalgia. And here's the good news: They are also *treatable* with the use of a fairly simple group of supplements, taken once a day.

This was exciting new information, and we have now completed the next phase of this research. In the original project, all patients received exactly the *same* supplements for six months. But now we wanted to answer a different question: If we treat these patients separately and individually, based on their unique, measured biochemistry and genetic information, can they get even better?

To test this hypothesis, we continued treating the same patients, and with the expertise of Dr. Amy Yasko, who measured their genetic information; Dr. Rich Van Konynenburg; and Dr. Tapan Audhya, the head of the Health Diagnostics and Research Laboratory, we formulated individual treatment programs unique to each patient. We based each treatment on the biochemical and genetic information that we had obtained from testing each patient, and we followed them for three additional months. We continued to test their chemistry and follow their clinical improvement with questionnaires.

What we discovered was that these patients *continued* to improve, particularly with the addition of Dr. Yasko's unique methylation treatment materials consisting of proprietary RNA preparations and trehalose. We saw continued and significant rises in glutathione and SAM, and with it, patients had various degrees of clinical improvement. Several patients, who had only reported 10 to 15 percent initial improvement, now told us they were 50 to 60 percent better. One patient, who had not worked in more than five years, was able to successfully resume full-time employment!

But that's not all. At the end of our program, based on research done by Sidney Baker, MD, with autistic children, we added one more therapeutic piece for nine patients. Dr. Baker had discovered several years ago, that if he treated autistic children who had elevated adenosine levels with acyclovir (an antiviral antibiotic with additional benefits to methylation chemistry), they improved. Well, nine of our patients, who had gotten better, but not achieved optimal results, still had elevated adenosine levels at the end of nine months of treatment. (Adenosine buildup strongly implies that the methylation cycle is not moving properly and adenosine is critical in the formation of ATP (adenosine triphosphate), which we require for energy.) So I offered them an additional two to three months of a trial of the medication acyclovir, 200 mg, five times daily, and all of them agreed to try it. The results: Eight of the nine patients reported an additional 20 percent improvement.

The upshot of all of this information is that now these patients who had experienced 30 to 60 percent improvement on our previous treatment program were now describing 60 to 90 percent improvement on completion of this study. From my perspective, there is no question that this represents a major new addition to our treatment options for these individuals.

Now you can see why I'm so excited about methylation chemistry and why I am so eager for you to understand even a little of it. For example, you might read this material and realize how important it is to raise low glutathione levels. The obvious question would be: "Why don't you just give these patients glutathione?" That has been tried by numerous investigators, using glutathione in every form available: oral, intravenous, transdermal, even rectal. Although these treatments produce some benefit, they don't last, so success is quite limited. It turns out that if the body is deficient in glutathione because it can't *make* it, giving it to the body in *any* form is merely a temporary fix (only hours, actually) and sends the body the wrong message. If the body *thinks* it has adequate glutathione, it stops making it, and that makes everything worse. So we have to restore the body's innate ability to *make* glutathione to achieve health. Our research results show that this is now possible.

I won't show you any more diagrams of how these cycles actually interact with other important cycles, most notably the ability to make the essential neurotransmitters serotonin and dopamine, which we explored in the previous chapter. As mentioned earlier, a good example of the importance of this chemistry is that our ability to make melatonin, essential for sleep, rests on our ability to *methylate* serotonin *into* melatonin. If this process is impaired, we can immediately see how sleep could be affected.

Although the chemistry we are discussing is complicated, the treatment is not. The use of a simplified methylation protocol, provided at the end of this chapter, has now been utilized by several physicians in hundreds of patients with excellent results, quite similar to mine. As this is a natural therapy, improvement is not immediate. While a few patients report some improvement within a few weeks, the average time it takes to begin to notice improvement is six weeks.

However, I must provide some words of warning. Although these natural materials have no known side effects, when they do work, they may dramatically improve the body's ability to process stored toxins. If that happens, toxins may be released into the system in amounts greater than the body's ability to deal with them, and these patients may initially get worse. Keep in mind that this is not a side effect; it reflects the fact that our treatment is working. These reactions are not rare. We have seen these reactions in up to 50 percent of our patients, varying from very mild (the usual reaction) to one that was quite severe. Usually, these reactions reflect an exacerbation of underlying symptoms, the most common being an increase in aches and pains and fatigue. A few have reported abdominal symptoms consisting of stomach cramping, constipation, or diarrhea. A few have reported headache. These symptoms have usually resolved within a few days, once we have decreased the dosage or changed the frequency of administration from nightly to every other day, every third day, or in rare cases, once a week. Once the body adjusts to the lighter dosage, we can usually get our patients up to the full dosage and see the full benefits.

Please do not take this warning lightly. I truly believe that these supplements should only be taken under the direction of a knowledgeable, experienced medical professional with training in this area. As they say on television: "Please, folks, don't try this at home."

Our research has recently been reviewed by Dr. Martin Pall, a biochemist from Washington State University who has published extensively on the biochemical underpinnings of chronic fatigue syndrome, who feels that the results of our study give further weight to his research on how imbalances in the nitric acid cycle also provide an excellent explanation for the underlying dysfunctional chemistry of chronic fatigue and fibromyalgia. (See Further Reading at the end of this chapter.)

## EDWARD'S STORY

*Edward's story not only describes benefits of methylation treatment, but in its complexity gives an excellent example of how these ideas come together to promote healing.*

Edward was a medical student who came to see me in his last year of training. He had been "reasonably functional" until eighteen months prior, when he experienced the onset of waves of nausea, severe fatigue, difficulties with mental concentration and focus, and numbness and tingling around his mouth and left hand. He had a complete evaluation by neurologists, gastroenterologists, and others. He did have adult-onset diabetes, which was carefully monitored. No real cause for his symptoms was uncovered by conventional testing, but Edward was obviously concerned as these symptoms seriously impaired his ability to function as a medical student.

Edward had read about Wilson's syndrome and found a local physician who started him on long-acting T3. On this he began to feel somewhat better, especially with his memory and concentration, but his energy didn't really improve. Other relevant components of his history included a severe bout of mononucleosis in college with a recurrence several years later, documented sleep apnea, and a slip on the ice in his second year of medical school, which injured his sacrum.

In response to measured low levels of DHEA and magnesium, bacterial pathogens in his GI tract, notably Klebsiella, and a visual contrast/FACT test that suggested neurotoxicity, we began treatment with DHEA, magnesium infusions, supplements for his bowel and digestion, transfer factors for the Epstein-Barr infection, and Welchol for presumed neurotoxicity. Osteopathic manipulation was also provided at each visit.

Edward improved somewhat on this regimen, but he was still so fatigued and mentally compromised that he was having difficulty completing the last few clinical rotations that would allow him to graduate from medical school. He was frightened that he would not be able to graduate and would not realize his dreams of becoming a physician. Since Edward was a compassionate and bright young man, this would indeed have been tragic.

An unusually severe setback after a viral infection suggested that his immune system was compromised by adrenal deficiency, and testing for this revealed it to be true. We started him on Cortef, and he began to improve again. After four months, he was still not well enough to function adequately at school, so we began the methylation protocol along with the use of D-ribose (a natural supplement of the sugar that is the backbone of DNA; deoxyribonucleic acid) for energy. Within two months, he was improved enough that he successfully completed his studies and graduated from medical school. He was still not convinced that he was well enough to begin his residency program (I shared his concerns in that regard), so we measured his methylation chemistry and despite taking our supplement protocol for three to four months, he still had profoundly low glutathione and folic acid levels (making us wonder how low it would have been had we tested him before beginning the protocol).

When we added new supplements to improve his methylation chemistry, he got much better and was able to begin his residency program as scheduled. He was very pleased that he was able to work long hours, but was still just "getting by." We measured his iodine levels and they were low, and when we added Iodoral treatment, he had another obvious improvement in his level of functioning. His tremors and numbness and tingling sensations were virtually gone, and his visual contrast/FACT testing had returned to normal. At his last visit he remarked that he felt better than he had in years, despite the long hours of work and training. He was able to go to social functions and needed less sleep and fewer naps. Working with Dr. Gene Shippen, a physician who has clarified the understanding of hormonal function, especially testosterone, Edward was able to improve his testosterone and growth hormone levels, which enabled him to complete his training and begin a promising medical career.

---

Edward's story gives us a nice example of how we can take a step-by-step approach to the treatment of these complex medical problems.

If we are patient and observant, we can figure out what we need to do to restore these compromised patients back to good health, and that, for me, is truly fulfilling.

I would like to point out that we have tried this protocol with several patients who have reported to us that they have been depressed since childhood, for no clear reason, and several have improved dramatically with its use. We have also used this protocol with patients that have autism, ADHD, and ADD, with clinical benefits in most cases. Those physicians who have been working with autism for some time (see Chapter 22) are well aware of how important methylation chemistry is for those children.

You can see that we have just scratched the surface of the importance of methylation chemistry in health and illness, and we are excited by the prospect of making great strides in this new area of study.

## FURTHER READING

Yasko, Amy. *The Puzzle of Autism: Putting It All Together.* Bethel, ME: Neurological Research Institute, 2006.

Nathan, Neil and Richard van Konynenburg. "Treatment Study of Patients with Chronic Fatigue and Fibromyalgia based on the Glutathione-Depletion Methylation Cycle Block Hypothesis." *Townsend Letter,* December 2011.

Pall, Martin. *Explaining "Unexplained Illnesses": Disease Paradigm for Chronic Fatigue Syndrome, Multiple Chemical Sensitivity, Fibromyalgia, Post-Traumatic Stress Disorder and Gulf War Syndrome.* Binghamton, NY: Harrington Park Press, 2007

# PART THREE

# New Approaches to the Relief of Pain

---

It would be a rare human being who had never experienced pain. Alas, it is an all-too-common part of our existence. For some fortunate individuals, pain is fleeting, minimal, and does not interfere with their day-to-day life. For others, pain becomes a lifelong struggle.

Part Three is devoted to an understanding of both acute and chronic pain. Like the rest of this book, it is not intended to present a comprehensive discussion of this subject; that could take volumes. Rather, it is my intent to describe the essentials of good pain diagnosis and treatment, and to single out a few specific treatments for discussion. To continue the theme of hope for those who have been told that nothing more can be done, I want to show how a different approach to diagnosis opens up whole new avenues of treatment that the reader may not have previously considered.

In our current medical system, part of the problem with evaluating pain is our emphasis on specialized care. Just recently I saw a young woman who had three different specialists—one for each area of her pain: her neck, her midback, and her lower back! I can only describe this as fragmented care, and unless someone is looking at the bigger picture, the treatments of one physician may unwittingly be in conflict with those of another physician.

Each specialist naturally puts an emphasis on his or her own perspective (often to the exclusion of other considerations). So for the evaluation of low back pain, we would not be surprised to find the neurologist and neurosurgeon focusing on the nerves or on structures that impinge on nerves. And we would expect the orthopedist to focus on the bone structure and spurs. And we would expect the rheumatologist to focus on the joints. And we would expect the chiropractor to focus on body alignment and structure.

In my world, where people with complicated problems turn up on my doorstep, pain is multifactorial. That is to say, my patients' pains are produced by a complex interaction involving not only the nerves, bones, joints, ligaments, tendons, and structural alignment (all of which interact with each other), but also include biochemical imbalances that produce persistent inflammation. Unless I can look at the whole picture, I, too, risk getting stuck using one perspective, and then it becomes unlikely that the problem can be accurately diagnosed or treated. Again, as stated throughout this book, diagnosis reigns supreme. My efforts, therefore, will go toward looking at this pain problem from as many different perspectives as I can bring to the table.

This section begins with an overview of how to look at pain in this way, with an emphasis on how a whole body area needs to be evaluated and treated. I will then attempt to persuade you that a different model for treating acute pain is needed in an attempt to prevent recurrent or chronic pain. I would like to share with you a research study I completed ten years ago in which we treated 250 consecutive cases of low back pain, and I hope this will clearly make my point.

Then I will discuss several treatments with which you may not be familiar: osteopathic craniosacral manipulation, prolotherapy, frequency specific microcurrent (FSM) treatment, and low energy neurofeedback stimulation (LENS). These discussions will hopefully show you that other approaches to managing pain do exist and may be helpful in providing relief for or curing your pain problem.

# CHAPTER 15

# Introduction to the Treatment of Pain

## A Pain in the Derriere

Perhaps the most common complaint that people express when they arrive in my office is that of pain. Low back pain, neck pain, shoulder pain, chest pain, abdominal pain, headache, and generalized pain (including fibromyalgia and arthritis) are of major concern for most of my patients, and the vast majority of them have already seen many other physicians and healthcare providers for consultation before they arrive at my office. The very fact that they have found my office makes it clear that they have not had a satisfactory diagnosis or treatment, so obviously we must begin there.

It is my impression that since these individuals have failed to improve with a wide variety of treatments, the single most frequent medical mistake in the treatment of pain is the lack of a clear diagnosis. Now this might seem obvious, but without a clear, concise understanding of the cause of a problem, how are we expected to formulate a viable treatment plan?

In the current language of pain specialists, when a patient presents with pain, we must search for the pain *generator*. Where, exactly, is this pain coming from? Let's take low back pain as an example—the commonest pain complaint seen by family physicians. When someone points to her lower back and says, "It hurts right here," that should be just the beginning of our evaluation. Regrettably, in conventional medicine, with the limited amount of time available to evaluate any medical problem thoroughly, hasty diagnoses are made. This often pressures the time-challenged doctor to an off-the-cuff diagnosis of mechanical low back pain for this particular patient, which is far too vague to be of use in formulating a treatment plan. The conventional approach for this "disease," as we will discuss in our next chapter, is the prescription of pain medication or muscle relaxants. The patient then takes her prescription medications, and if she is lucky, the pain will go away on its own. These medications are not specific for the treatment of our patient; after all, we have not defined the specific tissues that have been injured here. Pain relievers and muscle relaxants only buy us a little time in which the tissues may heal on their own, if they are able to heal at all. They treat the symptoms, not the cause.

If the pain doesn't go away promptly, the next medical step is usually to provide physical therapy. Again, if the patient is lucky, he will be referred to a physical therapist who will take the time to look for the pain generator and specifically treat it. If the therapist finds the injured tissue—muscles, joints, ligaments, tendons, discs, nerves, or a combination of these—the treatment can be properly directed. Unfortunately, many physical therapists are under the same time pressures as physicians, and they usually apply nonspecific remedies without a clear diagnosis, including ultrasound, neural stimulation, heat- or cold-based treatments, massage, and nonspecific stretching exercises. Again, with this type of treatment program, a lucky patient will see the pain resolve on its own. But if not, the patient may then be referred to a physiatrist (a rehabilitation specialist), orthopedist, neurosurgeon, neurologist, anesthesiologist, or pain specialist, who may or may not attempt to make a specific diagnosis to begin definitive treatment.

Most of my patients tell me that although they have had x-rays, CT and MRI scans, nerve conduction tests, and have seen multiple specialists, no one has actually touched the affected area to examine it. While this may sound harsh, this has been reported to me so frequently over the past twenty-five years that I have come to believe my patients. This oversight in examination has been observed by many pain specialists and represents a major problem in the medical care that our pain patients receive. As obvious as it seems, one cannot make a clear diagnosis with actually touching or palpating the injured tissues to look for the pain generator. (*Palpation* is simply the medical term we use to delineate the use of our hands in carefully examining a particular tissue of the body.) In the next chapter, we'll see that this problem has been compounded by the current medical belief that physicians *can't* make a clear diagnosis of what is causing the pain. So why should we even try?

## HENRY'S STORY

Henry was a prominent neurologist from Kansas who came to see me fifteen years ago with what he described as low back pain. For the previous five years, he had seen an array of his colleagues, including orthopedists and neurosurgeons, who had diagnosed a bulging disc in his lower back as the source of his pain. These specialists provided Henry with a variety of treatments. He underwent surgery to remove the disc, with no relief of his pain or symptoms. Multiple steroid injections into the lower back had provided no relief either. With the continuation of his pain, Henry became frustrated, and when a colleague mentioned to him that I might have a different approach, he came down for a visit.

When I asked Henry to describe his pain, he pointed to his right buttock and described a severe pain in that area, especially when he sat for too long. As he reflected on his symptoms, he recalled that this was actually his initial symptom, which really had not changed over this five-year period of time. This pain started in his right buttock and radiated down the back of his right leg to his calf, following the distribution of the sciatic nerve. When I examined him, he had no pain near or around the lower spine or sacroiliac joints. His pain could be reproduced by touching the right ischial tuberosity ("sitting bone"). The muscle directly above this region that spans the buttock, called the piriformis muscle, was in rather severe spasm (see Figure 15.1 on the following page).

The piriformis muscle is especially important when we evaluate patients who complain of sciatica, since the sciatic nerve often runs right through the body of this muscle. If that muscle tightens up or goes into spasm, it can pinch the sciatic nerve in a misguided effort to attempt to protect the nearby pain generator (in this case a bursitis of the ischial tuberosity, or sitting bone). In my experience, spasm of the piriformis muscle is by far the commonest cause of sciatica and is frequently over-

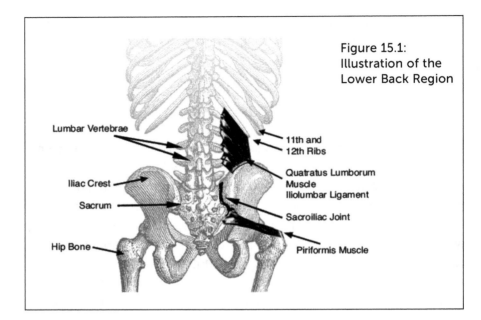

Figure 15.1:
Illustration of the
Lower Back Region

Lumbar Vertebrae

11th and
12th Ribs

Quatratus Lumborum
Muscle
Iliolumbar Ligament

Iliac Crest

Sacrum

Sacroiliac Joint

Hip Bone

Piriformis Muscle

looked as the source of sciatic symptoms; instead, most physicians focus their diagnostic efforts exclusively upon the lower lumbar spine. There is a bursa, or sac, which covers the ischial tuberosity to lubricate it and protect it from the friction of all the sitting we do. If that sac becomes inflamed, we call this an ischial tuberosity bursitis, which is just a fancy term for bursitis of the sitting bones.

I told Henry that I thought this was his diagnosis and that it could explain all of his symptoms. I offered him a simple injection of cortisone into the ischial tuberosity region, along with an injection of Marcaine, a long-acting local anesthetic, into the irritated trigger points of the piriformis muscle, which Henry accepted. We then followed these injections with a stretching of that muscle so that it could resume its normal resting length.

Having spent the past five years wrestling with this pain and looking exclusively at the lower spine as its cause, Henry was a bit skeptical that my treatments would work. No one had ever proposed this diagnosis to him, and neither had anyone ever examined his buttock before. I performed this simple procedure (which took all of three minutes) with his full cooperation, and for the first time in five years Henry reported imme-diate and complete relief of his pain. Still shaking his head and doubting that this would last, he discovered that this relief actually lasted for several weeks. He returned three weeks after his first visit for a second injection, and after that the pain disappeared completely and it never returned. Henry was a happy camper. He subsequently referred quite a few patients to my office for evaluation and treatment of their pain.

---

Henry's story emphasizes some of the points I have been trying to make. Despite the fact that Henry was a specialist and well aware of the various possible causes of lower back pain, he was so caught up in the conventional medical model that it somehow never occurred to him that he and his treating colleagues were on the wrong track. Even surgery had proven ineffective. The real problem was that no one had actually examined his area of pain. Once the pain generators had been identified, specific treatment could be provided, allowing healing to occur. Henry spent five years in pain and underwent unnec-essary surgery because this basic principle of medicine was not fol-lowed.

Our bodies are complicated, but if we study them, they usually make a great deal of sense. It is a cliché to say that everything is connected to everything else, but if we forget this simple fact, we are missing out on the full medical picture. The lower back, which we've been dis-cussing, is an excellent example of this. If we return our attention to Figure 15.1, it will illustrate for us the main players that affect this region:

The most common pain generator in the lower back, from my expe-rience, is an injury to the sacroiliac joint. People with these injuries usu-ally complain of pain directly over that joint. They may also complain of pain radiating down their leg, or pain over the lower back muscles, or pain in the lower rib cage on that side, or deep pain in their groin. How do we explain all of that? It's actually quite simple: We must understand the anatomical connections.

In Figure 15.1, you can see that there are several ways in which the body may try to manage sacroiliac joint pain: It may tighten up the piriformis muscle, as we discussed in Henry's story, which may pinch the sciatic nerve and cause pain to radiate down that leg. The piriformis muscle is paired with the psoas muscle that spans the front of the groin. If the piriformis muscle contracts or goes into spasm, so will the psoas muscle, which will cause pain in the groin area. Additionally, the muscle above the sacroiliac joint, the quadratus lumborum (the thick lower back muscle which most people think of as their main back muscle) may tighten up, with the same protective reflex. The quadratus lumborum, in turn, is attached to the lower rib cage just above it. Yanking tight on those ribs, the quadratus lumborum may pull on the ribs with enough force that it can jam the joints with which those ribs attach to the spine, and this sets off lower rib cage pain.

Treatment of this common form of lower back pain is based on an understanding of these muscular interactions. The patients' description of their pain areas leads us quickly to understand which part(s) of this system we need to focus on. If pain is radiating down the leg, we need to look at the piriformis muscle. If the pain is in the groin area in front, we need to examine the psoas muscle. If the pain is described in the lower rib cage area, we need to examine the quadratus lumborum muscle and the lower ribs. Often we need to examine *all* of these areas to clarify how they are interacting. Here's the important part: Once we have identified which tissues are producing our patient's pain, *we need to treat them all.* That is, we cannot just inject the sacroiliac joint if that is the main cause of pain, but we must also treat the jammed ribs and all of the associated muscles that are in spasm. Then the whole system can settle down and heal.

If we miss just one component of the problem, that component may not allow complete healing, and although the patient may initially improve, the symptoms will keep coming back. Our patients are often the perfect guides to what we may have missed. If we are really listening to them, they will tell us that though some of their symptoms have improved, they are left with different symptoms now. That description will point us to the next area that requires treatment.

I call this process *layering*. What hurts the patient most will get all of his or her attention. It's sort of like the old adage "The wheel that squeaks gets the grease." There may be other painful areas, but the worst one may be the only one that grabs the patient's awareness. If we remove that pain, often we find another pain below that. Sometimes people get frustrated by this and tell me the pain has "moved." Usually it hasn't actually *moved*. They are merely becoming aware of the next layer of pain, and now this can receive our full attention for healing. It usually doesn't take more than a few layer removals to provide substantial improvement or cure.

Now that you are aware of these basic principles, let us take a more detailed look at our treatment options for pain in the next chapter.

## FURTHER READING

Weiner, Richard S., ed, *Weiner's Pain Management: A Practical Guide for Physicians,* 7th edition, Informa Health Care, 2005.

For a more in-depth discussion about chronic pain, the reader may wish to view a free two-hour presentation given at the Mendocino Coast District Hospital that was filmed for public television and can be accessed at www.mcdh.org by going to its home page, then going to Health & Wellness, and then going to Videos on Demand.

# CHAPTER 16

# Can Chronic Pain Be Prevented?

---

## An Ounce of Prevention . . .

There exists in the current practice of medicine an odd prevailing misconception: Not only does acute pain not need to be treated aggressively, but the cause of acute pain cannot be accurately diagnosed; hence, even designing a treatment is futile. Some of you may think this is an exaggeration, but I can promise you it's not.

Dr. Richard A. Deyo, from the Oregon Health and Science University, has written extensively on this problem of diagnosis and treatment of pain. He asserts that "up to 85 percent of patients with low back pain cannot be given a definitive diagnosis because of the poor association among symptoms, pathological findings, and imaging results." The current accepted model for treatment of acute low back pain was developed by the Agency for Healthcare Research and Quality (AHRQ). This consensus organization has reviewed the available research in this field and has concluded that the initial assessment of patients with acute low back pain should focus on the detection of "red flags." These flags are time-honored findings and symptoms that suggest serious or life-threatening causes and include conditions in which spinal nerves are pinched or damaged. Red flags, according to the AHRQ, include bulging discs that impinge upon the nerves or spinal cord, metastatic cancers, or spinal stenosis (a bony narrowing of the spinal canal that compresses the spinal cord). If not diagnosed and treated promptly, we would all agree that our patients would be subject to significant harm. Red flags can also include the loss of bowel or bladder control, loss of sensation or strength in one or both extremities, or loss of reflexes. Medical practitioners, myself included, agree completely with the need for looking for and treating these red flags. However, when we understand that only 2 to 3 percent of patients show these particular symptoms, we realize that the vast majority of patients with back injury, who do not have red flags, will not receive that kind of attention.

In the absence of these red flags, the AHRQ has proposed that imaging studies and further testing of patients with acute low back pain are not usually helpful in the first four weeks following injury. They suggest that relief of discomfort can be accomplished most safely with nonprescription medication and/or spinal manipulation. Bed rest for more than four days is not recommended, and patients are encouraged to return to work or their normal daily activities as soon as possible. What this means is that if you are suffering from acute low back pain and you don't have one of these red flags, your doctor will probably tell you to take some ibuprofen or Tylenol and get back to work as soon as possible.

I have treated pain for many years, both acute and chronic, and this concept made little sense to me. More important, it did not fit with my own observations that a precise diagnosis of acute pain was entirely possible and essential to correct treatment. With exact, early, aggressive treatment, it was my impression that patients did quite well, and it was rare to see the onset of chronic pain afterward. Conventional medical wisdom says, "Statistics reveal that approximately 10 percent of patients with back pain complaints do not get better in four to six weeks," and "more than half the people who recover from a first episode of acute low back pain will have another episode within a few years. Their problems with back pain become chronic."

So in 1999, in order to delve deeper into this subject, I embarked on a research project. This entailed taking a part-time position with a clinic specializing in occupational medicine, a clinic that contracted with the largest employers in our area. What made this particularly relevant was that we were working with a captive audience: In these large companies, all of the injuries and pains sustained on the job had to be reported to the employer, and they had to come to us for evaluation and treatment. This gave us excellent access to follow-up care. I was assigned to evaluate only those severely injured patients who had suffered acute pain injuries and were not responding to our routine care. We evaluated and treated 250 consecutive patients with acute low back pain and another 100 consecutive patients with acute injuries to their neck, thoracic spine, and head areas. We kept careful records of our treatment results, including return-to-work data and whether these same patients came back to our clinic with recurrent symptoms within a three-year period. As we discuss the concepts of pain in this chapter, I will often refer to my experiences at this clinic.

Before I relate the results of that four-year study, let's start with trying to understand why conventional medicine does not believe in an accurate preliminary diagnosis. You may not like the answer, but it's simple: Most physicians are not trained to examine the musculoskeletal system with their hands, so they over-rely on x-rays, CTs, and MRIs to make their diagnosis. Unfortunately, in this area, these testing methods are a little crude. MRIs, for example, are unable to distinguish small but significant structural abnormalities of 2 millimeters or less. So for larger structural problems, like a protruding disc, they are excellent. But to detect a muscle that is in spasm or a slight spinal or joint abnormality, MRIs simply don't have the visual resolution to make the diagnosis. But our hands do.

Although I'm an M.D., I've been blessed with some wonderful osteopathic and chiropractic teachers who have taken the time to teach me how to feel for and treat these problems. With this information and hands-on treatment, we can make presumptive diagnoses about exactly where our patients' pain is coming from. We can then get clear feedback from their response to our treatment, which will further clarify whether our diagnosis is correct or not.

Here is a simple example. As mentioned in the last chapter, the most common acute low back injury in my experience is that of acute sacroiliac joint strain. First of all, the injured patient will point to those joints when she describes her pain, and when I examine her, I find that those areas are much more tender than the surrounding tissues. I can then inject the sacroiliac joints with a mixture of Marcaine (a long-acting local anesthetic) and cortisone (for longer relief of inflammation), and I find that if the diagnosis is correct, the patient reports immediate decrease in pain. Over several days, this pain decreases or disappears completely. To me, this is pretty good presumptive evidence that we did identify the source of pain and treat it correctly. In this way, we can systematically go over the entire area of pain and come up with a clear diagnosis. How the patient responds to the treatment makes it quite clear how accurate the diagnosis actually is.

Keep in mind that in an injured patient, it is not always that simple. The injured tissues are connected to other tissues, which may also be injured. We have to look at the whole picture. For example, in a patient with an injured sacroiliac joint on one side, the muscles that surround the injured joint usually tighten or go into spasm as the body attempts to protect that injured area. As we discussed in the previous chapter, the quadratus lumborum (the thick muscles on the sides of the lower back) tighten, pull on the lower ribs, and often "jam" them. All of this leads to pain in the lower rib cage area. The piriformis muscle across the buttock and its companion muscle, the psoas (in the front of the groin), also tighten to protect the area, and the pain may radiate into those areas as well. Commonly, the sciatic nerve runs through the piriformis muscle, and when that muscle contracts protectively, it literally *pinches* the sciatic nerve, causing pain to radiate down the patient's leg. So, we have to take all this into account and treat it all. Treating just the sacroiliac joint may not be sufficient. Figure 16.1 on the next page shows a posterior (back) view of this area and illustrates this relationship.

Take, for example, a badly injured worker with severe right-sided sacroiliac pain. He also experiences accompanying spasms of the piriformis, psoas, and quadratus lumborum muscles, as well as jammed ribs of the right lower rib cage. He will therefore present to us complaining of pain that is worse in the right sacroiliac joint area, but also radiates up into the right lower rib cage, down the right leg, and into the right groin. A comprehensive approach to treating this problem would include:

- An injection of the upper and lower poles of the right sacroiliac joint

- Osteopathic manipulation of the sacroiliac joint, especially if ilial rotation (a hip that is out of alignment) is present

- Release of the jammed ribs on the right side

- A muscular release of the spasm in the piriformis, quadratus lumborum, and psoas tissues

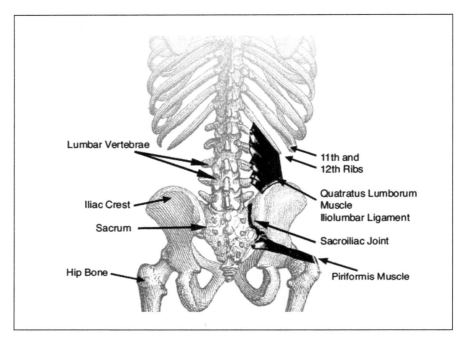

Figure 16.1: The Anatomy of the Quadratus and Piriformis Muscles
and Their Relationship to the Sacroiliac Joint

⊛ Trigger-point injections or myofascial release techniques and perhaps
the identification and treatment of other affected muscle groups, such
as the gluteus or tensor fascia lata

You can see that this would be a far cry from simply offering ibuprofen for four weeks and waiting to see if it worked or not. The exact
treatment, of course, would depend on the exact tissues that were found
to be injured by our careful evaluation. If my patient responds well to
the specific treatments I provide to those areas, it is a pretty safe bet
that those were indeed the injured tissues. This makes me quite certain
that a specific tissue diagnosis for low back injures is entirely possible,
and, in fact, *necessary* for correct treatment.

That was precisely our approach at the occupational medicine clinic
that I joined in 1999. Each patient was carefully evaluated and then
treated by me and a team of other healthcare providers, which included

another physician trained in osteopathic manipulation. Each injured area was treated with methods suited to the nature of that injury: injections, osteopathic manipulation, medication, physical therapy, and combinations of those modalities.

What did we learn through using these methods? Table 16.1 shows the discoveries we made about the nature of pain generators for those who presented to us with low back pain.

## TABLE 16.1: PAIN GENERATORS FOR ACUTE LOW BACK PAIN

### SOURCES OF PAIN IN 243 CONSECUTIVE PATIENTS

| | | | |
|---|---|---|---|
| Sacroiliac Joint | 80% | Quadratus Muscle | 20% |
| Piriformis Muscle | 21% | Rib Head Pain | 10% |

### OTHER MUSCLES (PSOAS, GLUTEUS)

| | | | |
|---|---|---|---|
| Ligament Injury | 6% | Greater Trochanteric Bursitis | 2% |
| Somatic Dysfunction | 4% | Sacrococcygeal Injury | 2% |
| Herniated Disc | 3.2% | Iliolumbar Ligament | 1.5% |
| Facet Joint | 3% | Chronic Low Back Pain (Non Specific) | 1% |
| Ilial Rotation | 3% | | |
| Ischial Tuberosity Bursitis | 2% | Spinal Stenosis | 0.5% |

If you total up the percentages in Table 16.1, it is clear that they are greater that 100 percent when summed. This is because, as I have been stressing, each patient often has more than one pain generator. You can see that injury to the sacroiliac joint was by far the most common injury component, and that a herniated disc, which is what most patients fear most, was only present 3.2 percent of the time. This percentage is compatible with most studies in the medical literature.

More important, we found that of our recently injured low back pain patients, of those whom we treated proactively, only 18 of 243 came back to the clinic with a recurrence of back pain over a three-year follow-up. This represents a reinjury rate of only 7.3 percent, whereas national statistics suggest that in people treated by the conventional, passive medical model, the re-injury rate is closer to 50 percent! This is quite significant, so much so that it suggests that our proactive approach to treating acute pain clearly prevented the majority of relapses.

We followed our patients for at least three years after their original injury, and only eight of them (3.7 percent) went on to develop chronic pain, whereas by national statistics, this should have been much higher. To be more specific, "statistics reveal that approximately 10 percent of patients with back pain complaints do not get better in four to six weeks" and that "more than half the people who recover from a first episode of acute low back pain will have another episode within a few years. Their problems with back pain become chronic." You can see that we clearly demonstrated a marked reduction in both recurrence of low back pain and the onset of chronic pain.

We also followed another 100 patients with other injury-related pains, including spinal injuries involving the cervical or neck area, thoracic or midback area, and injuries to the head. As you can see from Tables 16.2 and 16.3, the results suggest that most common bodily injuries respond well to our treatment process and also suggest that the diagnosis-based proactive treatment approach that I am advocating may not only improve the rapidity of healing, but also may prevent recurrent or chronic pain in most cases.

| TABLE 16.2 CONSECUTIVE ACUTELY INJURED PATIENTS (N=364) | | |
|---|---|---|
| **BODY AREA** | **REINJURY** | **CHRONIC** |
| Lower Back: 243 patients | 18 (7.4%) | 8 {3.2%) |
| Neck/Shoulder: 71 patients | 1 | 2 |
| Thoracic/Ribs: 39 patients | 6 | 1 |
| Head: 11 patients | 0 | 1 |
| Total: 364 patients | 25 (6.9%) | 12 (3.3%) |

### TABLE 16.3   ACUTE LOW BACK PAIN AGGRESSIVE TREATMENT—243 CONSECUTIVE PATIENTS

| | | |
|---|---|---|
| Reinjury | 18 patients | 7.4% |
| Chronic Pain | 8 patients | 3.2% |

We also looked at how quickly these people were able to return to work. Since we were working in an occupational medicine clinic, this was of great interest to the employers who paid us for our work. Table 16.4 below shows our findings.

### TABLE 16.4: TIME FROM ONSET OF SPINAL INJURY TO RESUMPTION OF PART-TIME AND FULL-TIME WORK

| RETURN-TO-WORK STATUS: | MODIFIED WORK | REGULAR WORK |
|---|---|---|
| Low Back Pain (n=243) | 3.8 days | 24.2 days |
| All Pain (n=364) | 3.5 days | 23.5 days |

Unfortunately, there are very few good statistics available that would allow us to compare our results with those of others who have treated injured workers with acute low back pain by different strategies. Although we don't have those numbers, I can say from my long years of work in this field that the return to modified work in an average of 3.8 days ("light duty") and the eventual resumption of regular work in an average of 24.2 days ("regular duty") was impressive to the employers with whom we worked. They were quite pleased with our results. Keep in mind that in this study we were only treating the most seriously injured patients, which makes these numbers look even better.

The costs of chronic pain are well documented in terms of personal and familial losses, with staggering financial losses for both the individual and society. Our study suggests that this new model of understanding acute pain may lead to a whole different approach to treatment, which, in most cases, may prevent the pain from recurring or becoming chronic. Now, doesn't that sound a lot better than taking ibuprofen for four weeks and just hoping the acute pain will resolve?

# FURTHER READING

Ashburn, Michael A., and Linda J. Rice, eds. *The Management of Pain.* New York: Churchill Livingstone, 1998.

Bigos, S. J., O. R. Bowyer, G. R. Braen, et al. *Acute Low Back Problems in Adults.* Clinical Practice Guideline No. 14 (AHCPR Publication No. 95-0642). Rockville, MD: American Health Care Policy and Research, 1994.

Deyo, Richard A. "Fads in the Treatment of Low Back Pain." *The New England Journal of Medicine* 325(14), 1991.

Spilzer, Walter O. *Scientific Approach to the Assessment and Management of Activity-related Spinal Disorders.* Philadelphia: Harper & Row, 1987.

# CHAPTER 17

# Manual Medicine: Osteopathic Manipulation and Craniosacral Therapy

## Lend Me a Hand

Let us explore the role of touch in healing. From my perspective, the act of making physical contact with another human being allows us to convey something that words cannot. A doctor's touch, well beyond words, may speak volumes about our concerns for and feelings about our patients. I find that many of my patients arrive in our office somewhat jaded, having experienced repeated medical visits that have not met their needs. They have spent a great deal of time and money looking for a cure, yet often they feel unheard, even hopeless. Many of their physicians have suggested that there's nothing wrong with them, implying that their problems are essentially psychological.

While trying to stay hopeful, many of these folks are probably expecting more of the same from me, too. They have heard lots of words, lots of jargon, lots of verbiage, and many promises that have gone unfulfilled. Surprisingly, despite hours and hours of office visits, most patients have rarely been touched or carefully examined by their doctors. So if my patient experiences pain in a particular area, I will make every effort to not only examine that area thoroughly at the first visit, but to begin the process of treating it with manipulation. I have found that being touched by someone who genuinely cares, especially when it leads to immediate (even if temporary) improvement, conveys more than all of my words ever could. The act of physical contact carries the possibility of breaking through communication barriers and establishing a relationship on a deeper level. This is an excellent way to begin a therapeutic alliance, and, alas, one often neglected by my profession.

Manual medicine has been around for thousands of years, and it exists in a bewildering variety of forms or styles. But it is not my intention to catalogue these in any detail here; rather, I will simply provide an overview of this field to give you a sense of what can be achieved when the healing capacities of human touch are harnessed. Manual medicine is defined separately by each therapeutic discipline that provides it. Hence, there are osteopathic, chiropractic, physical therapy, massage, Ayurvedic, Rolfing, myotherapy, Shiatsu, and countless other forms of treatment. As the name *manual medicine* implies, practitioners use part(s) of their body to change specific musculoskeletal imbalances in their patient. Practitioners typically use their hands, but elbows, feet, and other body parts can also be utilized. The basic idea is that structural problems can be influenced and treated by either directly or indirectly working upon them. By structure, I simply mean imbalances and dysfunctions of specific anatomical areas: muscles, tendons, ligaments, bones, joints, connective tissues, and nerves.

Let's say you wake up in the morning and you've somehow slept "wrong" on your pillow. Now you've got a "crick" in your neck—it doesn't turn or rotate normally, and it hurts. As the morning moves along, you notice not only pain in the neck area, with restricted motion of your neck, but a headache and pain and tension in your shoulders. What should you do? If you sought conventional medical attention, you might be told you have a muscle spasm, which would be the correct medical diagnosis, and you'd probably be given pain medication or a muscle relaxant to take. After several days, your pain would probably go away slowly on its own. But if you were aware of the benefits of manual medicine and sought out that form of treatment, you would find a more specific and speedier form of relief. That "crick" in your neck is probably caused by a cervical vertebrae that is just a bit "out of place," and the resultant spasm of the neck muscles is your body's attempt to protect that painful area. By "adjusting" your neck, or putting that vertebra back into alignment, the neck muscles no longer have anything to protect, and your muscles can return to normal much more quickly.

My first introduction to manipulation came early in my career when

I had the privilege of working with Stan Weisenberg, a wonderful chiropractor, who shared my office space. While I noticed that my medication-treated patients took seven to ten days to get better, Stan's patients were getting better within a day or two, following his manipulative treatment of their necks and shoulders. So I begged him to teach me how to do it. Although we were friends, the climate of distrust between physicians and chiropractors in the early 1970s was such that Stan later confessed to me that he had to get up some courage to teach me; he was concerned that I might somehow view his work negatively. The opposite was true. I was astonished to observe how he could restore patients to health with carefully orchestrated treatment, and I began to learn how to manipulate necks and lower backs. It soon became obvious that my patients were now getting better much more quickly, and I started studying other types of manipulative medicine as well.

Stan and I had a mutual teacher of Reichian therapy (not to be confused with Reiki, which is a form of energy treatment) who encouraged me to study osteopathic craniosacral manipulation. This was a branch of osteopathy to which they, as chiropractors, did not have access as it was taught only to doctors of osteopathy (D.O.s), physicians (M.D.s), and dentists.

So, in 1975, I went to Colorado Springs to spend a very intense week with a roomful of superb healers, who kindly and gently began the process of instructing me. It is hard to convey how presumptuous my presence in that class was at the time: I had very, very little manipulative training and knowledge; in fact, I didn't even know what an osteopath was. I had no idea that they were physicians trained just as rigorously as I had been, but that they had also studied the art of manipulation in the service of healing. What I did recognize at that first course was that these physicians were really good at what they did. I saw them do things with their hands that I had never dreamt possible. They opened up doors that completely changed my life.

The most fascinating concept of that initial experience was to learn that the cranial bones were not fused together throughout life, as my medical teaching had suggested, but that these bones were designed from birth to move and to literally "breathe." Of course, this motion is exquisitely minute, but I was taught how to perceive it and work with it to restore normal motion in the bones, which translated into improved motion of the tissues to which the bones are attached.

When I left Colorado Springs, I was unsure about how useful this information would be, or how well I could apply it. A week after my return to practice, I would see a patient who would clarify this for me. I was working in the emergency room of our local hospital, and a young boy came in who had been playing shortstop in a Little League game. A ball had been hit to him and took a bad hop, striking him sharply in the left jaw. He immediately noticed loss of hearing from his right ear and severe pain, tingling, and numbness of his right jaw. Had I not taken this course in craniosacral manipulation, I would have assumed some vague mechanism of injury and told the family to go home and be patient, hoping that his injury would somehow wear off by itself over time. Instead, with my newfound knowledge, I could clearly see how the force of the injury to his left jaw had been transmitted into his right temporomandibular (jaw) joint and "jammed" his temporal bone, affecting his ear and causing all of his symptoms (see Figure 17.1).

Using craniosacral therapy, I simply freed up his right temporal bone and jaw joint. My treatment consisted of inserting one gloved finger into the boy's mouth, while I held onto his cheekbone on the same side with my other hand. Inside his mouth, I applied a tiny amount of upward traction on his sphenoid bone, which I accessed by resting my little finger behind his upper teeth, while I rotated his cheek bone away from its "jammed" position. I then changed the position of my fingers inside his mouth so that I could grasp his right lower jaw, and I applied gentle traction downward, freeing up his jaw joint. Within seconds, all of his symptoms disappeared. I was amazed (as was the boy and his family). More important, I realized how useful this information was going to be and launched into an even deeper study and appreciation of this whole field.

Since my own study of manual medicine has been primarily osteopathic, I'd like to focus on the principles of this form of treatment. The first principle of osteopathic treatment, as enunciated by founder A. T. Still in the late 1800s, is "The rule of the artery is supreme." Initially, this might sound a little vague or obscure, but let's explore it a bit more. Dr. Still was referring to the fact that anything that compresses or

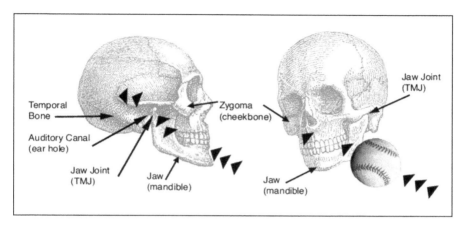

**Figure 17.1: Diagram Illustrating the Mechanism of Injury**

restricts arterial blood flow in any way prevents oxygen from reaching the tissues supplied by the arteries. These tissues would include muscles, tendons, ligaments, bones, nerves, and organs. In essence, every tissue must receive free, unrestricted arterial blood flow for optimal functioning. By identifying with precision all areas of restriction, a trained osteopath can restore blood flow to those tissues and powerfully influence the restoration of health.

Dr. Still was referring to more than just arteries, however. His rule actually applies to all areas of flow within the body. Anything that restricts those flows—whether that flow is arterial, venous, lymphatic, neuronal, respiratory, or even energetic—needs to be identified and freed up. The free, unrestricted flow of all fluids in the body is thus one important and often overlooked aspect of health. We can expand that concept to include the ability of the body to freely expand and contract and move (which even includes free flow on a cellular or biochemical level) as one part of the goal of good health. This rule of "the artery is supreme" is indeed a profound concept, and when applied toward healing, it is well worthy of in-depth study.

Identifying restrictions in flow of arterial and other fluids then becomes an important part of the healing process and is an essential feature of osteopathic treatment. Once again, we are talking about clear diagnosis, which can lead to a very specific, precise treatment plan.

Whether we find a tight muscle, fascial strain (the fascia is the connective tissue that surrounds the muscles), a bone or joint restricted in its motion, or a nerve that is impinged upon by other structures, we can find multiple methods of relieving these restrictions using the wide variety of manipulative techniques available to us.

I believe manual medicine is an underutilized component of healing. While conventional medicine barely recognizes the existence of this branch of healing, for centuries people have been aware that physical touch can relieve pain, and they have sought those with skills in this area for comfort and healing—and often received the help they were looking for.

## HEIDI'S STORY

Heidi was a thirty-seven-year-old woman who had been suffering with constant daily pain located over her right cheek area and across the bridge of her nose, involving the front of her face below her nose and her upper and lower teeth. This had progressed over a seven-year period to include frequent headaches across her temples.

By the time I saw her, Heidi had already seen many excellent neurologists, neurosurgeons, and several other physicians who had prescribed every medication under the sun. None of the medications really helped, and many of them caused her significant side effects. She had received a steroid injection to a branch of the right maxillary nerve, under her right cheek, about a year previously. That area was still numb and tingling, and the injection had not relieved any of her pain. She also described persistent pain in her low back and sacral areas. As we explored the cause of these symptoms in detail, Heidi really didn't know what had set it off those many years ago. The pain had become debilitating, and the constant wrestling with it had left her exhausted, making it difficult for her to take care of her children and husband and function well in her career as a therapist.

When I evaluated Heidi from a craniosacral perspective, she had marked restriction of motion of her whole cranial mechanism, especially the facial bones, and a significant restriction of motion of her sacrum as well. (There is a direct anatomical connection between the sacrum and the base of the skull so that these are very closely related; restriction of one can easily affect the other.) Treatments involved freeing up her neck and shoulders and upper ribs (tightness in those areas affects the cranial structures) and extensive work with the cranial and facial bones. This included gentle traction upon all of the cranial bones, along with work inside her mouth to free up the cheek, sinus, and jaw restrictions, as well as work upon her sacrum and lower back tissues. As I treated her osteopathically every two weeks in all these areas, she slowly improved. Within four months of treatment, she reported to me that she was 85 percent better. She would go whole days where she experienced almost no pain at all. She also experienced improved energy and sleep and marked relief from her back pain. After a few more months of osteopathic treatments, she described 95 percent improvement.

Interestingly, after our first few treatments Heidi recalled having injured herself on two occasions from falls she had incurred. In one fall she struck her right cheekbone, and in the other she had fallen directly upon her face, particularly affecting both her upper and lower teeth. These areas that she injured were exactly the areas that were now causing her so much pain. The process of freeing up injured tissues often releases the memory of how the injury occurred. It is fascinating to observe how frequently practitioners of osteopathic manipulation find this to occur when we treat with manual medicine. Patients are often surprised that they have somehow forgotten important parts of their history that help to explain their symptoms. We refer to this phenomenon as tissue memory, which reflects the fact that the memories are actually contained in the injured tissues and not simply in the mind, as most people believe. Furthermore, emotions that may be connected to this injury are often bound up in the myofascial tissues themselves. The process of treating those injured tissues often brings forth the emotions that have been held in those tissues so that they can be expressed. This emotional release often greatly contributes to the healing process.

I believe that Heidi would not have recovered without this form of treatment. Time alone (seven years' worth in this case) did not cure her. Precise identification of the cause(s) of her pain was essential to her healing. With the benefit of that precise diagnosis, we had the tools we needed to be of service.

Nothing is as simple as it sounds, unfortunately. For those of you who are thinking of seeking a qualified practitioner of craniosacral therapy, please be aware that there are several schools that teach this procedure and that there are significant differences between these schools.

The original information on this subject was discovered and thoroughly researched by William Garland Sutherland, D.O., beginning in the early 1900s. Dr. Sutherland single-handedly put a curriculum together over many decades. Therefore, the osteopathic craniosacral teachings have the longest history and usage, and are the most detailed and sophisticated approaches to correcting craniosacral imbalances, but have only been taught to D.O.s, M.D.s, and dentists. An osteopathic physician named John Upledger simplified Sutherland's osteopathic teachings and has made them available to chiropractors, physical therapists, massage therapists, and lay healers. By its basic nature, Upledger's revised methods can help with simple structural problems, but any complicated or sensitive structural problems may require the services of the full osteopathic training program for healing. In fact, if applied incorrectly, or in a heavy-handed fashion by those not properly trained, one can actually jam the sutures (which are the defined boundaries between cranial bones) and do harm to the membrane and fluid physiology, injuring or damaging the patient. So be sure to delve into the training background of an individual who claims to do this form of therapy. It may sound like a bit of a cliché, but all craniosacral practitioners are not created equal, and that principle can be expanded to include virtually any treatment technique that you might seek. No practitioner should be offended by your inquiries into their training background; that information should be offered freely and comfortably.

There is a structural—physical—component in virtually every pain problem we see in our office. Many practitioners of medicine focus on the emotional components of pain, unfortunately conveying to the patient that they believe the problem is in the patient's head. Far too often, a careful evaluation of long-injured tissues, which include muscles, fascia, joints, bones, and nerves, has not been performed. So if you have a long-standing pain problem, this is an area of treatment that you may well wish to explore.

## FURTHER READING

Copland-Griffiths, Michael. *Dynamic Chiropractic Today: The Complete and Authoritative Guide to This Major Therapy*. San Francisco: Harper-Collins, 1991.

Magoun, Harold. *Osteopathy in the Cranial Field*. Kirksville, MO: The Journal Printing Company, 1966.

Prudden, Bonnie. *Pain Erasure*. New York: Ballantine Books, 1980.

Rolf, Ida. *Rolfing: The Integration of Human Structures*. New York: Harper & Row, 1977.

Travell, Janet, and David Simons. *Myofascial Pain and Dysfunction: The Trigger Point Manual*. Baltimore, MD: Williams and Wilkins, 1983.

Upledger, John E., and Jon Vredevoogd. *Craniosacral Therapy*. Seattle, WA: Eastland Press, 1983.

To find a practitioner of craniosacral manipulation in your area, visit the Cranial Academy's website at www.cranialacademy.com, or call (317) 594-0411 for a referral.

## CHAPTER 18

# Prolotherapy, FSM, and LENS

---

## No Pain, No Gain: An Introduction to Exciting New Ways to Treat Pain

In this chapter I discuss three methods for treating pain that may be unfamiliar to you. These are three of the most useful techniques that I have found to be effective in the treatment of pain (and other conditions), when conventional methods have not been helpful.

### PROLOTEHERAPY

In addition to craniosacral therapy and other forms of manual medicine, another highly underutilized treatment for chronic pain conditions is prolotherapy (formerly sclerotherapy). In prolotherapy, a mildly irritating solution is injected into injured or dysfunctional ligaments or tendons of the body, so that at the site of that injection we are intentionally creating an inflammatory reaction in those tissues. This, in turn, stimulates the natural healing forces of the body to bring new cells, called *fibroblasts*, into the inflamed tissues to deal with this inflammatory process. (The *prolo* in *prolotherapy* is a shortened form of the word *proliferate*, a clear description of what is occurring here on a cellular and tissue level.) The fibroblasts grow, or *proliferate*, in the ligaments we have injected. The growth of these fibroblasts creates a thicker, stronger ligament or tendinous insertion, which, as we shall soon see, directly promotes healing. Studies have been done in rabbits showing that ligaments can potentially grow 40 percent stronger by using this treatment. Humans respond well to this method, and it is the only method I know of in which a ligament can truly be strengthened.

Muscles, of course, can be strengthened by a wide variety of exercises. But ligaments, as they are an entirely different type of tissue, do not respond to the kinds of treatments so useful for muscles. The good news is that we now have, through prolotherapy, a way to heal damaged ligaments.

You may not be aware of how essential ligaments are in all joint functioning. The integrity of every joint in the body is created by and composed of ligaments. When a ligament becomes stretched or damaged, it is no longer capable of holding the joint together properly. Frictional forces start to wear away the smooth cartilage surfaces that cover the opposing bones that create the joint. Thus, the process of arthritis begins. When this erosion of cartilage becomes severe, we call it bone-on-bone, meaning that the cartilage has worn away so completely that the bones are now rubbing against each other. In a normal joint, the bones and the cartilage that covers them are held apart by the tight ligaments, allowing the lubricating fluid in the joint space to keep these tissues healthy.

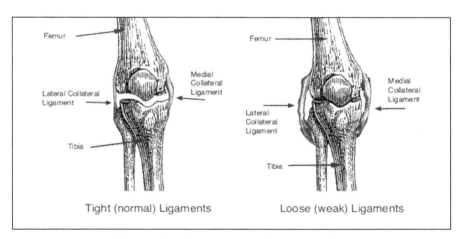

Figure 18.1: Structure of the Knee Joint

Let's take a look at the knee joint, depicted in Figure 18.1, for a clearer description of this process.

On the left we see a normal joint with tight ligaments that hold the joint spaces apart. Since we usually associate tightness with pain and strain, it's important to appreciate that this is the normal tension in the ligament and is essential to its functioning. If the ligaments become weak, as in the illustration on the right, the joint space collapses and the bones start to rub against each other, eventually creating an arthritic condition.

If we can stimulate these weakened ligaments to tighten, we can literally start to pull apart the bones that have collapsed into the joint space, thereby re-creating the normal joint space and normalizing the joint function. As long as the damage has not gone on for too long, we have the wonderful possibility of treating the wear and tear on our joints that would eventually become full-blown arthritis by using prolotherapy. It allows us to put off, sometimes indefinitely, the need for surgery or joint replacement, and it markedly improves or reduces arthritic joint pain.

Virtually any joint can be treated with prolotherapy. Let's take, for example, one of the most commonly injured joints: the sacroiliac joint. This joint is located in the lower back area between the sacrum (the thick triangle of bone at the base of the spine) and the two hip bones, which are medically referred to as the *ilia,* hence the technical term *sacroiliac.* Often people refer to this area as their hips, but technically that is not correct; the hip refers to the joint between the *femur* (the lower leg bone) and the *acetabulum* (the area in the pelvis to which it attaches). Look at Figure 16.1 again (on page 190) to refresh your memory about these anatomical relationships.

Lower back injuries frequently involve damage to the sacroiliac ligaments, and often patients are told by those proficient in manipulative medicine that their hip is "out of place." While this term is not used in conventional medicine, it is actually often correct. The weakened ligament caused by injury allows the whole ilium, or hip, to rotate around, usually making one leg longer than the other. This is fairly easy to diagnose. When these injured sacroiliac joints are treated repeatedly by manipulation but the hip won't stay in place, the ligaments have most likely been damaged. The use of prolotherapy in this instance can be exceedingly helpful.

Here is a brief description of the process involved in providing prolotherapy: While a variety of injection materials can be used, most often we employ a dextrose (sugar) solution of 12.5 percent or more, often coupled with a weak solution of phenol (an acidic compound) and perhaps sodium morrhuate (a fish oil) in sterile form. These materials act as irritants to the ligaments and cause the injected body areas to become inflamed and start producing fibroblasts. You might be surprised that dextrose can irritate the body, as it is a natural substance. It is true that dilute doses of dextrose don't have an inflammatory or stimulatory effect, but once the concentration gets to 12.5 percent or more, it can take on a new role and be effective in this capacity.

We inject this solution into the ligaments we wish to stimulate, a procedure that will be different for each joint of the body. The number of treatments, which can be given every two to four weeks, differs depending on the size and area of the ligaments or tendon areas that need to be stimulated. For example, an elbow problem, which most often would reflect what is commonly called *tennis elbow,* might respond to just two or three treatments. A shoulder or ankle problem usually responds to three treatments. Lower back and knee areas, which have a much larger ligamentous component, usually require six treatments or more to provide healing.

Once the materials have been injected, I urge my patients not to use any anti-inflammatory medications, including aspirin, Aleve, ibuprofen in its many forms (including Advil and Motrin), or Celebrex, for the entire duration of the treatment program. If pain medication is needed, Tylenol (acetaminophen) or a specific, stronger pain medication can be prescribed. We recommend that patients avoid ice or heat for the first few days after injections are provided, as ice may diminish the inflammatory process we are trying to create, and heat may exacerbate it to the point that the patient may suffer needlessly.

It is very important that the physician providing these injections is also trained in manipulative medicine. It is vital that when these tissues tighten up, they tighten up into the correct anatomical position. We encourage patients to use the area that we have injected as much as possible after the injections, as that helps the tissues to heal in the correct position for proper functioning.

## KRISTINA'S STORY

Kristina was a nineteen-year-old woman referred to me by a local physiatrist (a medical doctor who specializes in physical rehabilitation) who had tried for several years to get her hip to stay in place using manual medicine. He could get her hip into place, but no matter how hard he tried, it just wouldn't stay there. This physiatrist was familiar with the potential benefits of prolotherapy, and he recommended her to me for treatment. After explaining the process to Kristina and her family, I proceeded with the injections. After four treatments, each involving multiple injections into the ligaments covering the sacroiliac joints, her back held in place nicely. After years of persistent, debilitating low back pain, she became pain free for about a year.

It would be wonderful if this was the conclusion of the story in the form of a happy ending (there is one—hold on), but after a year Kristina developed severe migraine headaches, which seemed to have been set off by orthodontic procedures including the use of braces and spacers. Her orthodontist told her that her migraine headaches could not possibly have been caused by tightening her braces. Unfortunately, in my experience, this can indeed happen, and all too frequently. He referred Kristina to a neurologist who provided a variety of medications for the headaches. None of these medications worked very well and actually caused some severely limiting side effects, including mental fogginess, fatigue, and even more headaches, all of which interfered with Kristina's ability to cope with schoolwork.

Eventually I put this all together and sent her to another dentist who specialized in using bracing techniques that incorporated knowledge of craniosacral mechanics (see Chapter 17). With this dentist's help, Kristina's migraines improved dramatically. However, during this time, her hips began to go out again and would not stay in place, even though we'd gotten them to do so for the whole year previous. But I found that if I could get her jaw back into alignment, my hip adjustments, along with a single additional prolotherapy treatment, now held. The ways in which certain areas of the body relate to other areas in completely unsuspected patterns is truly fascinating. Kristina has essentially been well now for several years, without the need for additional osteopathic manipulation or prolotherapy.

---

Kristina's case is one in which the combination of prolotherapy and creative manipulative medicine resulted in a healing that had eluded her for many years.

I believe that we're going to see a lot more prolotherapy usage in the future. In the past several years, new research has revealed that much of what we used to call tendonitis is actually *tendonosis*. These words may seem similar, but they encompass very different understandings of the mechanical causes for pain. *Tendonitis* refers to an inflammatory condition of the tendon. For many years we have treated all inflamed and tender tendons with anti-inflammatory medication and steroid injections with the presumed diagnosis of tendonitis. We have known for quite some time that repeated steroid injections may actually weaken the tendons even further, and while these treatments help some patients, they often do not last and need to be repeated to the point where they become counterproductive. New research shows that these tendons are really not inflamed, but damaged. Having such damaged tendons is referred to diagnostically as *tendonosis,* which means that some of the fibers of the tendons are actually weakened and torn where they insert into the bone.

This new understanding of this common diagnosis provides us with an innovative rationale for treatment and explains why our old treatment didn't always work very well. To heal damaged, torn tendon-insertions, prolotherapy is a much more logical approach. In fact, it is much more useful than steroid injections and works far better over the long haul. By injecting these damaged fibers and using prolotherapy to stimulate the body to lay down new fibroblasts, we create a thicker, stronger tendon. This enables us not only to heal these tissues, but to create a stronger tissue, one that would have been rendered weak by steroid injections.

Over the past four years, a new form of prolotherapy has entered the therapeutic scene, which is called *platelet rich plasma* (PRP) *prolotherapy.* The areas that are injected are identical to those used previously, but *what* is injected here is a solution made from the patients' own blood. Prior to the injection, 20 cc to 60 cc of an individual's blood is drawn and spun down in a special centrifuge that allows us to separate out a fraction of the blood, which is, as the name implies, especially rich in platelets, as well as protein growth factors such as platelet-derived growth factors, transforming growth factors, vascular endothelial growth factors, and epithelial growth factors. Since the materials we are injecting here are made from the patient's own blood, we know that what we are using is compatible with that individual's chemistry. We then inject this material as we would our regular prolotherapy solutions. PRP appears to be much more effective in speeding up the strengthening process of these ligaments and tendons, probably because we are using concentrated, completely natural materials so that fewer injections can be used with equivalent or better results. PRP has also been found to be effective in improving the speed of wound healing.

## MY STORY

Approximately twelve years ago, while playing basketball with my son, I jumped up with my right arm fully extended in an attempt to block his shot and experienced a pain so intense that it literally dropped me to my knees. On reflection, I recalled that I'd had some twinges of pain in that shoulder for several years, but nothing prepared me for that moment. After that initial commanding shoulder pain, things eased up a bit, but then slowly and insidiously they became worse and worse. I was still able to work with that shoulder, experiencing moderate but tolerable amounts of pain, but I couldn't completely lift my arm.

Over the next six months, I saw several of the finest osteopathic physicians I knew, and each treated me graciously. But it made no difference. I could no longer sleep on my right side, but the most frustrating part was that I couldn't put my arm around my wife as we sat on the couch to watch television or read. That is what really motivated me to get treatment.

I eventually ran into an old friend, a wonderful osteopathic physician and practitioner of prolotherapy in Columbia, Missouri, named Larry Bader. When I visited Larry, I finally received an explanation for my pain that made sense to me. He described my injury as a "weakening of the shoulder capsule," a diagnosis with which I was not familiar. Larry smiled, noting that he hadn't been either until he'd experienced the same symptoms several years before. Essentially, the weakened ligaments of my shoulder capsule had allowed the joint structures to collapse upon themselves, permitting the supraspinatus tendon, one of the main tendons of the rotator cuff, to rub against the acromion, a nubbin of bone projecting downward from the scapula (shoulder blade). This is what was causing my shoulder symptoms. I have learned, subsequently, that this is actually quite a common condition, one often missed by specialists.

So I drove the three hours to Colombia, Missouri, for my three prolotherapy treatments, spaced about a month apart. While moderately painful, the injections were certainly tolerable, and I was sore for only a few days afterward. Treatment did not interfere with my ability to work. After the third treatment, it was clear that my pain was gone, and I could sleep on my shoulder again. But I still had a somewhat frozen shoulder, and I still could not lift my arm past shoulder level toward my head. I then received several treatments by a skilled physical therapist, which freed up my shoulder, and by working and exercising that shoulder I was able to achieve complete range of motion. I have not had a lick of pain or difficulty with my shoulder in the ensuing twelve years since I received my prolotherapy injections. Had I not done prolotherapy, I am fairly certain that this condition would eventually have deteriorated into a rotator cuff problem, which would have required surgery.

---

Here is one more story to illustrate the potential benefits of prolotherapy. It's about yet another patient who was told that joint replacement was the only possible treatment for her symptoms.

## BETTY'S STORY

I first saw Betty in 2000, when she was sixty-one. She was concerned about a wide variety of medical problems including generalized joint pains, chronic fatigue, dizziness, hypoglycemia, psoriasis, and a recurring rectal fissure. In short, she presented to us with the typical kinds of problems that I see in my office on a daily basis. Using the Big Six/ Little Six approach outlined in this book, I uncovered and treated thyroid problems, adrenal deficiencies, bowel dysbiosis, and allergy troubles that soon led to a marked improvement in her health. She was quite happy with the excellent improvement.

By late 2001, however, the deterioration of Betty's right knee joint became her central problem. Her orthopedic surgeon had recently performed arthroscopy for that knee, but she described the results of that procedure as disappointing. She was now informed by her surgeon that her right knee joint was bone-on-bone, meaning that there was no cartilage left in the knee to protect the joint. He told her in no uncertain terms that the only hope left for her would be to undergo total knee replacement.

As she was still a relatively young woman, she began to read up on prolotherapy and became intrigued with the possibility of this treatment for her knee. When she discovered that I could provide that service, we began treatments in early 2002. Since her knee damage was more extensive than most of my patients, it took ten prolotherapy injection sessions to produce the desired results. Betty was delighted that her pain was virtually gone: She could now walk up and down stairs without difficulty and resume the game of golf, which she had been unable to play for several years.

Seven years later, Betty has required no additional prolotherapy treatments and she continues to do well. She is thrilled to have avoided knee replacement surgery for so many years, and although we cannot be certain that this surgery will never be necessary, there is no sign currently that she is anywhere near that possibility.

---

Like Betty, I have often found that many patients who have been told, "There's nothing more we can do for you," have responded beautifully to prolotherapy and had much or all of their pain relieved. Please keep in mind that this is not a panacea for the treatment of all pain. It is specifically designed to treat pain that is caused by weakened or damaged ligaments and tendons. But as you can see, when used properly, it can be of enormous healing benefit.

## FREQUENCY SPECIFIC MICROCURRENT (FSM)

More than ten years ago, Carolyn McMakin, D.C., from Portland, Oregon, was working with a group of people with fibromyalgia using a new technology she had developed called *frequency specific microcurrent* (FSM). All of these patients shared the history of having had a significant whiplash-type injury that preceded the onset of their fibromyalgia, and on physical examination, all had especially reactive lower extremity (knee jerk) reflexes compared to those of their upper extremities, which suggested that they may have had a persistent inflammation in their spinal cord. Dr. McMakin had just refined her microcurrent device, which was capable of providing a specific electrical frequency that could remove inflammation through one electrical channel, and direct that energy to the spinal cord via a second channel. She noted immediate improvement in the majority of her patients, with cures of greater than 50 percent and significant improvement in almost everyone treated with the use of this device alone. By "cure" I mean complete resolution of all of the symptoms of fibromyalgia, which include not only migratory joint pains, but also fatigue, insomnia, and cognitive impairment.

Even more impressive, when she studied some of the biochemical markers for inflammation in these patients, including the interleukins, tumor necrosis factor, cytokines, endorphins, and cortisol, she was able to document 20-fold decreases in these inflammatory chemical markers and 20-fold increases in endorphins and cortisol in just a ninety-minute treatment! While the names of these markers may seem obscure, what Dr. McMakin's work really demonstrates is the ability of this FSM device to profoundly and quickly decrease inflammation and pain in nerve tissue. In a sense, the process represents a rebooting of the nervous system, allowing a system that has essentially been stuck on overdrive to return to normal functioning. This is nothing short of remarkable.

For the first time, we now have a treatment modality capable of removing inflammation from the spinal cord (and nerves and other tissues), which gives us an effective tool to help those patients whose fibromyalgia has been caused by spinal trauma. Dr. McMakin also gives us a new diagnostic label for this condition, which she calls cervical trauma fibromyalgia.

Since becoming familiar with this technology, I have personally treated over two dozen patients with cervical trauma fibromyalgia using FSM and have seen them respond dramatically. The treatment process is simple: patients are hooked up to this machine, which is fondly referred to as the "Blue Box" because of its distinctive color. The device is connected to the patient by electrical wires that are attached to electrically conductive graphite gloves, which are wrapped in towels that have been heated by warm water, and these are placed around the patient's neck and feet. Dr. McMakin has put together a comprehensive list of frequencies that relate to both specific tissues and physiological impairments, which are taught to prospective practitioners at several courses. The correct electrical frequencies, which are determined by the patient's physiology and confirmed by how the individual's muscles respond to those specific frequencies are then applied, while the patient lies back on a comfortable table, and we see how they respond. Whenever possible, at our first visit, I try to provide an hour or more treatment time as a diagnostic tool. For those with this cervical trauma fibromyalgia, response is immediate—meaning that at the completion of our treatment they report a 50 percent to 80 percent reduction in their pain levels, thus letting us know that this may be a major contributing component in their healing.

While this may be the most dramatic example of medical benefits from FSM, I would quickly add that it is a superb tool to treat virtually any form of inflammation, including those involving muscles, tendons, ligaments, fascia, organs, and nerves. In one case I have seen FSM shrink the size of a huge thyroid goiter in literally minutes. As with all new and exciting modalities, I suspect we have just scratched the surface of its potential in healing.

## LOW-ENERGY NEUROFEEDBACK SYSTEM (LENS)

Another new and exciting medical breakthrough is that of the low-energy neurofeedback system, or the LENS. Biofeedback has been used for many years, in different forms, to help improve body functioning. Most of that biofeedback has involved giving back information about a biological function (muscle tension, temperature, blood pressure, or brain waves) back to the patient so that he or she can slowly learn to alter that information. It is well documented that this form of treatment can help individuals to relax, lower their blood pressure, treat migraine headaches and pain, and to change brain functioning in ADHD, depression, and cognitive impairment.

What makes the LENS unique is that the patient does not have to be aware of the information being processed, and they do not need to cooperate with learning a new skill, which can be very difficult for someone with cognitive impairment. A sensor is attached to each ear and another to the scalp. No needles are used. The information detected by the sensors is fed (via an EEG device) into a computer that analyzes the brain waves from twenty-one different locations in the brain, a procedure referred to as brain mapping. The resonant, always-changing feedback into the computer through the EEG device is then conveyed back to the scalp where the brain can detect and recognize the feedback signals. This feedback, which is not volitional on the part of the patient, allows the brain waves to be, in a sense, redirected, creating a literal rebooting of the nervous system. For example, just last month, a patient of mine who had been very worried about her cognitive decline (she was concerned that this was Alzheimer's dementia and that she would never get better) who also had Lyme disease was treated with her second session of the LENS. Within moments of her treatment she was delighted to discover that her mind was much clearer and her thinking had improved, along with her memory. This shift not only held, but continued to improve with subsequent treatments.

This is especially helpful in those individuals who are unable to think clearly because their brains have been damaged or affected by toxins or infections. Most notably this includes people with traumatic brain injury (TBI), ADD, ADHD, Asperger's syndrome, autism, bipolar disorder, chemotherapy- or chemically induced cognitive impairment, anxiety, depression, epilepsy, stroke, Tourette's (tic) disorder, Lyme disease, post-traumatic stress disorder (PTSD), multiple sclerosis, Parkinson's disease, and early-stage Alzheimer's disease. What all of these conditions share, when uncomplicated by other medical issues, are variants of one fundamental process—how the brain tries to cope with actual or potential brain irritability—even though these conditions may present differently in different individuals because of the enormous variety in the way each person's brain develops.

Dr. Len Ochs, who developed the LENS process, believes that the inability to think clearly is partly the effect of the medical condition, but also the result of how the brain attempts to cope with actual or even anticipated brain irritability. Brain irritability can be caused by injury, chemical or heavy metal toxicity, or infections. The brain seems to try to deal with the spread of this electrical irritability by both chemically dampening that activity (suppression) or creating firewalls across both the surface of the brain and within the tissues of the brain to prevent those irritable signals from spreading. While these processes are natural, they interfere with the kinds of communication and connections the brain needs to function properly. Some people can recover from the presence of this altered neurochemistry when the brain puts out the "all clear" signal that the danger has passed. However, some people cannot refresh their neurochemistry or reboot the connections in their brains, and they may remain functionally impaired for life.

The LENS, using profoundly weak but precisely directed signals to the skin, appears to catch the brain's attention to allow it to interrupt its repetitive but nonproductive attempts to block its own communications, so it can resume more normal functioning.

Since discovering the LENS process, we have found it to be a superb and safe tool for people whose brain fog and cognitive impairment do not allow them to function properly. As an example: A young man came to our clinic just this year, having been in a serious motor vehicle accident several years ago in which he sustained a brain injury requiring hospitalization for a coma lasting several weeks. This resulted in his experience of prolonged exhaustion and the loss of his ability to think clearly or to express himself, which led to intense depression and mood swings, and his fear that he would never recover. Within two months of starting the LENS treatment he reported 60 to 70 percent improvement, after having made little to no progress over the previous two years. Depression and mood swings were gone, now, his energy had improved and he was able to think much more clearly, enough so that he started college classes again.

Of particular value to us in our work with Lyme disease is that many of those individuals have residual neurological deficits that continue even when the Lyme disease has been essentially cured. These symptoms include dystonias (odd, writhing, uncontrollable motions of the arms and legs), seizures, tics, and spasms. For some time we have felt that the nervous system, postinfection, was "stuck" in a pattern it didn't know how to correct. Kitty's first-person account below shows how the LENS was instrumental in reversing her residual neurological impairment and helping restore normalcy in the face of severe impairment.

## KITTY'S STORY

"In February, 2008, I had been hiking with a friend and my dogs came home with ticks. We found eight ticks in all, and most were still attached, but we also found a couple of engorged specimens crawling on the hardwood floors. A few weeks later, I came down with a flu that refused to go away. I didn't give it much thought until my chiropractor expressed concern about Lyme disease and rec-ommended that I be tested. I happened to choose a Lyme-literate physician who also tested me for Babesia (a parasite, also transmitted by ticks, that can cause a malaria-like illness). After five months of antibiotics and Mepron, I was worse than ever. I couldn't eat, I couldn't sleep, and I could barely get to the bathroom with my walker. I was in constant pain and my body was twitching and contorting in a most bizarre fashion. So I decided to get a second opinion.

"Although the second opinion was the same as the first, the method of treat-ment changed, and I slowly gained weight and strength. The neurological symp-toms waxed and waned, but I did not yet experience the symptoms of psychological disturbance and intense depression described in Lyme journals. I was still experiencing purpose, hope, and peace through all of the challenges I had faced to that point.

"In 2010 all this changed. As I regained my physical strength, something shifted and I suddenly began to lose my mind. I was familiar with odd sensations running through my body, but now, as my body buzzed and warbled, I couldn't reason my way through it. I found myself inseparably connected to a woman who threw temper tantrums and heard voices moan under her house all day long. I could not get her to behave. My body twisted and contorted like never before. I knew that hope was there, but couldn't reach it anymore. Why was I connected to this crazy woman who made absolutely no sense? Watching her terrified me.

"At this juncture, one of my doctors referred me to Dr. Neil Nathan. He quickly became a key member of my Lyme treatment team and also treated me for Bartonella (a bacterial infection transmitted by ticks, other insects and cats). When Dr. Nathan first suggested the LENS, I hesitated. But he assured me that within a few treatments we would know if it was a good fit for me, so the financial risk was low. I then met with an experienced LENS practitioner who endured the Lyme journey herself. Soon after my treatments began, the veil that separated me from reality lifted. My balance improved, my constant nausea abated, and I started thinking more clearly.

"The LENS also helped control my seizure activity, relieve Herx symptoms (the intense reactions that occur when the bacteria are killed and the toxins are released into the body), and aid in my recovery from chemical exposure. When I am exposed to certain fragrances my body shuts down. I can breathe and blink, but I often have to fight to stay conscious. Before LENS, I was given IVs and multiple shots to help pull me out. Although this made it possible for me to sit in a wheelchair, I faced a long process of recovery with each setback. On one occasion, I was heading to a LENS appointment when I was exposed to a common laundry detergent that repeatedly caused me problems. My LENS practitioner was confident that the LENS could help. So, with some great effort I was maneuvered into her treatment chair. You cannot imagine my delight as I watched my body respond. By the end of the session, I had regained full use of my arms and legs. Not only could I speak and hold my head up, but I could walk and laugh again.

"The LENS continues to pull me out of the ditch when I need it and helps keep my head above water. Even though my crazy sensitivities and responses cause me to take it slow, I'm able to tolerate antibiotics and other antimicrobials a little better. I can drive again and go out in public now. I am grateful for this noninvasive treatment that has made it possible for me to resume more of a normal life while being successfully treated for Lyme disease."

I hope that you will find this introduction to these exciting approaches for the relief of pain and the improvement in cognitive functioning will be of great value in your journey toward healing.

## FURTHER READING

Cyriax, J H., and P J. Cyriax. *Cyriax's Illustrated Manual of Orthopaedic Medicine.* 2nd ed. Oxford: Butterworth/Heinemann, 1993.

Dorman, Thomas A., and Thomas H. Ravin. *Diagnosis and Injection Techniques in Orthopedic Medicine.* New York: Lippincott Williams & Wilkins, 1991.

Hackett, George S. *Ligament and Tendon Relaxation Treated by Prolotherapy.* 3rd ed. Springfield, IL: C. C. Thomas, 1991.

Larsen, Stephen, *The Healing Power of Neurofeedback: The Revolutionary LENS Technique for Restoring Optimal Brain Function.* Rochester, Vermont: Healing Arts Press, 2006.

McMakin, Carolyn R., *Frequency Specific Microcurrent in Pain Management.* Philadelphia, PA: Churchill Livingston (Elsevier), 2011

# PART FOUR

# Other Concepts and Treatments for Those with Chronic Illnesses

I've always intended for this book to be one of hope, a resource people can turn to in their search for the next helpful step. Out of the many, many integrative and alternative treatments and concepts available, I am selecting just a few subjects for additional discussion. These subjects are chosen for their potential importance for many of those who are suffering from chronic illness.

Countless individuals have atherosclerosis and the subsequent blockages of vital arteries, including the coronary arteries that supply the heart with blood, the carotid arteries that supply the brain with blood, and the peripheral arteries that supply the extremities with blood. Statistically, this is the most common cause of death in America. For those people who have not benefited sufficiently from conventional approaches, the use of chelation therapy may be just what the doctor ordered. Chapter 19 provides a discussion of this underused treatment.

Cancer is the second most common cause of death in our society, and, when advanced, can be a serious source of suffering for patients and their families. Alternative concepts and approaches for the treatment of cancer are presented in Chapter 20. With the marked rise in autoimmune illnesses, clearly related to dysfunction of the immune system, this is a good place to include a discussion of the treatment options for these conditions.

With all chronic conditions, sleep difficulties become a major stumbling block on the path to healing. Unless the body can obtain adequate rest, it simply can't recharge its batteries, and everything gets worse. In Chapter 21 I will address this important area, from an overall perspective, and then more specifically look at the common presentations of sleep apnea and its recently identified cousin, UARS (upper airway resistance syndrome).

Finally, the current epidemic of autism is a frightening subject for all new parents. In Chapter 11 I will bring to your attention the exciting and effective new approaches to understanding and treating autism. The treatment programs that have evolved for autism are a kind of microcosm for many of the subjects that form the basis of this book: food allergy, heavy metal toxicity, chronic candidiasis, and methylation chemistry imbalances. Our discussion of autism will emphasize how helpful this entire approach can be for addressing the biochemical underpinnings of chronic illness.

# CHAPTER 19

# A Primer on Chelation

---

## The Bind That Ties

M uch is written about chelation, and as with any controversial therapy, much of this information is prone to misunderstanding and strong opinion. Since the primary use of chelation is for treating arterial blockage from atherosclerosis, most of the objections to its use come from cardiologists. They believe that there is inadequate scientific evidence to confirm its value, while ignoring the existence of medical books entirely devoted to providing this evidence. As this conflicting information brings us to a bit of an impasse, let us explore this subject in more detail.

The word *chelation* simply means "to bind," coming from the root word, *chela,* which is Greek for "claw." In general, the materials being bound are minerals, especially toxic heavy metals such as mercury, lead, aluminum, cadmium, tin, and arsenic, among others. Usually, when laypeople talk about chelation, they are referring to the use of ethylene diamine tetra-acetic acid (EDTA) chelation. This is by far the most common form of chelation currently in use, and it utilizes the chelating agent EDTA to bind to heavy metals, especially lead, to pull them out of the body. EDTA binds more tightly to the metals than body tissues do. The body then eliminates the EDTA with the heavy metal attached, moving it through the kidneys and out of the body through the urine. This has long been recognized by conventional medicine as the treatment of choice for lead toxicity.

EDTA chelation first became available during World War II, when it was used to detoxify workers who had excessive exposure to lead-based paints, most commonly from their work in the shipyards, where large quantities of these paints would be sprayed without adequate ventilation. It was discovered, however, that several workers with coronary artery obstruction (angina), had significant relief of their heart symptoms when their lead toxicity was treated with EDTA intravenously. Astute physicians who observed this wondered if EDTA might successfully treat other patients with coronary arterial blockages, and to their surprise it did. This launched the concept of "chelation" treatments in the management of arterial blockage from cholesterol plaques.

An EDTA treatment is fairly simple. We mix up a sterile intravenous infusion bag that contains an exact amount of EDTA, one that is calculated by precise measurement of the patient's kidney function. Added to the EDTA are magnesium and usually additional materials that may include small amounts of heparin, potassium, sodium bicarbonate, procaine, vitamin C, and B vitamins. The main limiting factor as to how much EDTA can be given is how well the kidneys work. Before we start the chelation process, we obtain a twenty-four-hour urine collection coupled with a blood test that measures the creatinine clearance, considered the most accurate way to define how well the kidneys are filtering. A normal creatinine clearance is 80 cc/min to 120 cc/min. Any value that falls lower than this range indicates that the dosage of EDTA must be decreased so as not to overload the kidneys.

With the correct amount of materials, the person receives a series of twenty or more intravenous sessions, initially given once or twice per week. Each of these sessions lasts an average of three hours. Depending on clinical response, these treatments can continue until maximum improvement has occurred. What I typically see is that patients report fewer episodes of angina, less shortness of breath, improved energy, an overall improvement in their sense of well-being, lower blood pressure, and a decreased need for their cardiac medications.

At this point, we continue these intravenous treatments once every four to six weeks, as maintenance therapy, indefinitely. We have discovered that if the patient goes more than six months without receiving treatments, some of the benefits may disappear. For the relief of arterial blockages, I have personally seen fairly dramatic improvements in cardiac function, along with improved blood flow to the feet and legs from the relief of peripheral artery disease, and improved blood flow to the brain from relief of carotid blockages. These treatments are *safe*. In thirty years of providing thousands of these treatments, I've only observed a few minor side effects and nothing negative of any significance. That's not a bad track record, especially when we compare it to the conventional medical alternative of surgery. There are well-known, life-threatening complications of cardiac catheterization (in which balloons or stents are inserted) and surgery (such as bypass operations), and the benefits may be short-lived. Balloon angioplasties often do not last for long, and stents often become blocked. While I don't believe that chelation is for everyone, it is certainly an option for many. Let's put it this way: If I were personally diagnosed with any arterial blockage, I would get chelated before I would undergo cardiac catheterization or surgery.

As previously noted, chelation has been accompanied by intense controversy over the years. Most conventional physicians believe that this treatment has no validity whatsoever and should never be attempted. Other physicians who have observed the effects of these treatments are convinced that this is a safe and effective process. As I write these words, several large, ongoing clinical trials are in place, attempting to clarify the answer to these important questions. Some observers of this controversy boil it down to economics: When you can charge $40,000 for a highly technical cardiac procedure, why would you consider an approach that only nets you $2,000? Many people who have benefited greatly from this procedure have been quick to point out this discrepancy.

## DUNCAN'S STORY

Duncan first came to me when he was fifty-nine, in February 1997. He expressed his major concern very succinctly at our first visit: "I've got plugged-up arteries." Duncan related a long history of coronary artery disease that began in 1980, when he underwent a six-vessel bypass procedure. Then, in 1992, he had a second four-vessel procedure performed. He had become concerned with increasing symptoms of shortness of breath and chest tightness and with the results of an angiogram performed in December 1996 that showed 100 percent occlusion of his right coronary artery grafts and 75 to 90 percent occlusion of a second graft area. His cardiologist did not feel that he could reach that area of occlusion with a balloon or stent, and medications were not effective in improving his condition.

I began treating Duncan with EDTA chelation therapy, which involved twenty initial treatments and one treatment monthly thereafter. Duncan did extremely well with his program, noting marked improvement clinically, which was confirmed a year later on a follow-up angiogram. By the time he had completed the first ten treatments, he was no longer short of breath, no longer had chest pain, and was able to go to work all day with increased stamina and energy. His cardiologist was amazed by his improvement, but as is usually the case, was loathe to attribute this improvement to Duncan's chelational efforts.

Duncan did very well on this program, and he was able to continue full-time work for many years until his expected retirement at age sixty-five. He continued his treatments but did have a minor setback in 2007, when he needed the placement of two stents by his cardiologist. Years later, continuing his chelation treatments, Duncan continues to be active and healthy and is convinced that he would not be alive today had he not undergone this form of treatment. I suspect that is true. Although his cardiologist still doubts the benefit of his chelation treatments, he has often commented to Duncan that his impressive improvement is baffling and admits that it cannot be explained by conventional medical concepts. But Duncan just smiles and shakes his head; he has no intention of stopping this treatment that has proven so effective.

---

Again, what I often hear from conventional cardiologists is that there is no evidence of chelation's efficacy, but there is actually quite a bit of medical literature that reviews this topic. It depends, really, on what you choose to read. If you don't read any alternative medical sources, it's not surprising that you're not aware of this evidence and information. Much of this book discusses what I would consider cutting-edge medical concepts, so my own opinions are based more on what I have observed and seen with my own eyes rather than on the opinions of others. But please don't misunderstand. I highly esteem the opinions of my colleagues and will take the time to listen closely to what they have to say. However, often those opinions are based on a theoretical understanding of an idea, rather than direct hands-on experience with a particular treatment, and it is the latter that I especially value.

There is a clear distinction between theory and practice. Theories are nice, but how real, live people respond to treatments is what I really care about. That's the frontline of medical practice: helping patients. If you spend any time around a group of patients who have had chelation treatments, it is difficult to walk away from that experience without being impressed. It is commonplace for patients to receive these three-hour infusions in small groups in my office, and listening to them recount their experiences to each other makes it difficult to discard the consistently reported benefits. After thirty years of administering these treatments, I am convinced that they have great value, and I would esti-mate that 80 percent of the patients who have participated would agree.

## MELVIN'S STORY

Sixty-two-year-old Melvin first came to my office in 2003. He had undergone a five-vessel bypass procedure fifteen years previously and originally came to me for persistent left-side numbness and tingling over his entire left rib cage, radi-ating up into his left neck area. He had been extensively evaluated in several medical centers, but with no explanation for his symptoms. I eventually treated him with osteopathic manipulation, which over the course of many months resulted in virtually complete resolution of his symptoms.

But in January 2005, Melvin had a mild heart attack and had several stents placed by his cardiologist. He was placed on the medication Plavix (an antiplatelet drug used to prevent blood clots), which is standard procedure fol-lowing the placements of stents. The side effects of the Plavix were almost worse than the cardiac symptoms: severe, sudden episodes of esophageal spasm that kept putting Melvin in the hospital for evaluation. And the stents just kept on coming. Over the next year, Melvin had ten procedures with the placement of a total of fifteen stents, performed on an almost monthly basis!

Despite the fact that he lived a considerable distance from our office, I encouraged Melvin to begin chelation to avert the continuation of this process. He agreed, although the procedure was difficult for him, as he experienced the very unusual side effect of shaking for several hours after each infusion. But as long as he continued his chelation, he was able to do well and did not require additional stents. After approximately eight months of treatments, he elected to stop them, and within a few months he was back requiring stenting procedures at an alarming frequency. The benefits of chelation therapy in this case seemed very clear to me, and they did to Melvin, as well.

---

The second most common form of chelation is the one we use for mercury toxicity (see Chapter 10). It is only recently that we learned how to accurately measure chronic mercury exposure, and as most physicians and dentists don't seem to realize that this is much of a problem, they do not address it. I can understand why dentists would rather not accept this information, as they have been placing mercury amalgam fillings in our mouths for over sixty years. It would be difficult for any health practitioner to believe that what he or she has been doing could be harmful, but as our knowledge grows, for many patients this seems to be the case.

There are three major sources of mercury exposure: fish ingestion, the emissions from coal-burning plants, and leakage from our dental amalgam fillings. Of those, most experts working in this field believe that the amalgams represent our greatest exposure. This does not mean that you have to run out and get your fillings removed today. Just because you have them doesn't mean they've leaked mercury into your body. Removing fillings is expensive and painful, and it should be done in a very specific manner by specially trained dentists so that additional toxicity does not occur. If you have reasons to suspect mercury toxicity (see the list of symptoms in Chapter 10), get your mercury levels checked using the DMPS challenge test, described later in this chapter.

## NATALIE'S STORY

Natalie, at sixty years of age, presented to my office in 2007. She was concerned about her hormonal balance, having been on Prempro and other synthetic hormones previously. However, those materials did not agree with her, and since she was hearing a great deal about the potential toxicities of synthetic hormones, she was fearful of taking them. Natalie was especially worried about her memory, focus, and concentration, and had particular concerns about her ability to work with numbers. This was of great importance in her job as a bank supervisor. For many years, she had prided herself on her ability to keep track of multiple columns of numbers at will, and now she could barely keep a column straight. Natalie also reported a significant drop in energy, as well as hair loss and emotional instability. She could now cry at the drop of a hat and felt at times like she could "tear someone's head off."

Upon examination, I found that Natalie had a low DHEA level, so I started her on 25 mg DHEA each morning. We discovered, as well, that she had low levels of estrogen and progesterone, so we provided a small dose of those bioidentical hormones. Both low estrogen and low DHEA levels are often associated with decreased cognitive function, but even after using those supplements for several months, Natalie was only slightly better from a cognitive standpoint. While her energy was quite a bit better and her mood much improved, her biggest concern was still that she couldn't think clearly, especially in working with numbers.

When I performed the DMPS challenge test (for mercury toxicity), I found she had a significant elevation in her mercury levels. We then began a monthly series of DMPS intravenous treatments, providing a total of eight. This was followed by the use of oral DMSA for the next year and then by the removal of her mercury amalgam fillings by a knowledgeable biological dentist. Slowly and steadily, within that year, the vast majority of her cognitive facilities returned, she was now functioning much better at work and at home, and she was very pleased with her improvement. Natalie feels that she is back to her old self, and that improvement has held steady over the ensuing years.

––––––––––––––––

Mercury tends to accumulate in our tissues, especially in the brain, and once there, it binds so strongly to those tissues that it is hard to remove. Time alone does very little. We have learned that simply measuring mercury levels in the blood, urine, hair, or stool will not reveal its presence, as it is tightly bound to body tissues. In order to diagnose it, therefore, we have to use a chelating agent (in this case DMPS is considered the best by most authorities on the subject). The chelator (DMPS) binds tighter to the mercury than it does to body tissues and pulls it out through the kidneys. By providing an infusion of intravenous DMPS over fifteen minutes, and then collecting the patient's urine for twenty-four hours and sending it out to our reference laboratory for analysis, we can get an accurate estimate of the mercury content of the tissues. This is an elegant and accurate test, and it, too, is cutting-edge medicine.

Still, experts are not in complete agreement about the best way to measure and treat mercury toxicity. What I have discussed represents a consensus of our current thinking, but some physicians prefer an oral chelator called DMSA, and others use the medication penicillamine. The point of this discussion is not to provide the definitive answer about how to measure and treat mercury toxicity, but rather to suggest that this is an often missed diagnosis. It should be considered as a possible contributing factor for anyone who is ill for whom no clear answers to the cause of their illness have been uncovered, especially when their symptoms include cognitive impairment, headaches, and unusual neurological presentations.

We have discovered several hundred patients with mercury toxicity, and most of them would tell you that removing the mercury has been of great benefit in their recovery. Newer ways of administering chelating materials have been proposed recently, including via oral, rectal, and transdermal administration. Unfortunately, there is very little evidence to suggest that these routes of administration work anywhere near as well as the intravenous materials. People are thrilled to hear that they might not need to take the expensive and time-consuming IVs, but at this time I cannot recommend the oral or other newer forms as an acceptable alternative.

## FURTHER READING

Cranton, Elmer M. *Bypassing Bypass Surgery: Chelation Therapy: A Nonsurgical Treatment for Reversing Arteriosclerosis, Improving Blocked Circulation, and Slowing the Aging Process.* Charlottesville. VA: Hampton Roads, 2001.

McDonagh, E. W. and C. J. Rudolph. *A Collection of Published Papers Showing the Efficacy of EDTA Chelation Therapy.* Gladstone, MD: McDonagh Medical Center, 1991.

# CHAPTER 20

# The Importance of Sleep in Healing

## Perchance to dream . . . ah, there's the rub

For the past twenty years, my dear friend Jacob Teitelbaum, M.D., has been emphasizing the importance of sleep in the healing process for those who have chronic fatigue syndrome and fibromyalgia. It seems intuitively obvious that if you cannot recharge the batteries properly, you won't have sufficient energy. And, in fact, the vast majority of my patients with chronic illness report a wide variety of sleep disturbances.

When sleep *is* disturbed, this sets off another vicious spiral of disability, at times making it unclear whether the illness is causing insomnia or whether lack of sleep is contributing to the illness. Both are true. My patients get so frustrated with how awful they feel when they are not getting adequate rest that they become fixated on paying detailed attention to every aspect of their sleeping process. As you might expect, this just makes it worse, because sleep requires relaxation as a central component to its initiation. The more worried you become that you might not be able to sleep, the more your thoughts and fears interfere with sleep, making this a kind of self-fulfilling prophecy. If we add unpredictable levels of pain to this equation, addressing these issues becomes a vital part of our treatment program. As pain has been addressed already, I merely want to emphasize that it may need to be taken into account so that it does not prevent our patients from achieving their much-needed sleep.

For sleep to become restorative, a lot of complicated biochemistry has to weave together seamlessly. It helps to understand a number of factors about sleep, so that we can address sleep problems in a more specific and helpful fashion.

## SLEEP ARCHITECTURE

While we often think of sleep as one experience ("I slept well" or "I didn't sleep at all"), when sleepers were studied carefully with EEGs (machines that measure brain wave activity), four stages of sleep were identified: REM (rapid eye movement) sleep, in which most of our dreaming occurs; and three stages of NREM (non-rapid eye movement) sleep. These NREM stages are called N1, N2, and N3 for short and represent a spectrum from wakefulness to deep sleep that can be measured by polysomnography (a special test used during sleep studies) in specialized sleep labs.

Stage N1 refers to the transition of the brain from alpha waves to theta waves and is often called *drowsy sleep*. During this phase, sudden twitches and jerks may occur, and the individual loses some muscle tone and most conscious awareness.

In Stage N2, muscular activity decreases further and conscious awareness of the external environment disappears.

In Stage N3, called *deep or slow-wave sleep,* we see an increase in delta waves. During this deep sleep stage we may see night terrors, enuresis (bed-wetting), and sleepwalking in susceptible individuals.

Each sleep cycle lasts from 90 to 110 minutes on average, and each stage may have a distinct purpose. The transitions from one stage to another must be in balance or one might experience sleep that results in loss of consciousness but is not restorative—meaning it *looks* like you have slept for a reasonably long time, but you still feel exhausted.

The reason it is important to understand this is that treatments must not only allow you to sleep longer, but more deeply (that is, more stage N3 sleep). Many sleeping pills and tranquilizers in common use (e.g., Dalmane, Halcion, and Valium) may actually worsen the quality of sleep by increasing the amount of light, stage N2 sleep and decreasing deep, stage N3 sleep.

## SLEEP CHEMISTRY

Basic sleep chemistry involves an understanding that *getting* to sleep requires an adequate amount of a neurotransmitter called *gamma-aminobutyric acid* (GABA), but *staying* asleep requires sufficient amounts of serotonin (see Chapter 13). With this realization we can begin to prepare to help a disordered sleep process. If an individual reports that they can get to sleep without difficulty, but wake up repeatedly throughout the night and cannot get back to sleep, we can focus our treatments around helping them to improve their serotonin levels.

Strategies to do this include the use of natural materials that build up serotonin, such as 5-HTP (5-hydroxy-tryptophan) and tyrosine, which we reviewed in Chapter 13. Other natural remedies that may address this specifically include St. John's wort (300 to 900 mg/day) and SAMe (200 to 800 mg/day). Medications can be targeted to do this as well, using small doses of amitriptyline (10 to 20 mg at bedtime), doxepin (10 to 20 mg at bedtime), or trazodone (25 to 50 mg at bedtime). These are not habit-forming or addictive and, in the tiny amounts used to improve sleep, are usually well-tolerated with minimal or no side effects.

To stimulate the GABA receptors, natural supplements include valerian root, passion flower, and kava kava. Medications include the benzodiazepines such as Valium, Ativan, and Xanax, and the related, more specific sleeping medications Ambien and Restoril. These medications do have addictive potential, and we need to weigh the potential risks of habituating someone to these medications against the need for sleep. As described previously, some of these medications may deprive us of the deep stage of sleep so essential for rejuvenation and we must take that into consideration here. Lunesta can be used for this context as well, with less risk of addiction, and Benadryl in various forms is available over the counter for this same purpose.

We have found other supplements with less specifically targeted usage, such as eclonia cava (Fibroboost), and melatonin—an important biochemical piece to the sleep process (1 to 3 mg at bedtime), may be of benefit here. I would caution you to always check with your healthcare provider to be certain that none of these suggestions could cause any detrimental effects for you; I would also strongly encourage you to realize that each of these supplements should be tried in small doses, one at a time, so that improvements in sleep will be noticeable. If a supplement does not provide obvious benefit, there is no reason to continue taking it. Combinations of supplements are feasible, but again, only under the direction of a knowledgeable healthcare provider.

Another important biochemical component of sleep is cortisol. As we discussed in Chapter 3, there is a natural cycle to the body's production of this hormone. It is made while we sleep, so that our peak levels occur when we first get up in the morning, and levels drop as evening approaches. There is a master clock in the brain that responds to light and regulates hormone production, especially melatonin and cortisol. The area of the brain that is supposed to respond properly to this information is the hypothalamus, which regulates the pituitary gland. We know this to be compromised in almost all chronic illness. This may result in a reversal of these natural cycles, resulting in too little cortisol during the day, when you need it, and too much at night, when it causes blood sugar levels to drop and wakes you up, often between 2 and 4 AM. To manage this, remember that eating high-protein food at bedtime (and avoiding carbohydrates) helps to stabilize blood sugar levels through the night (see Chapter 9). Since stress is the critical factor resulting in an overstimulation of the adrenal gland, relaxational strategies may be very helpful here. Learning meditation, yoga, tai chi, biofeedback, or the use of relaxation tapes are safe methods of improving this aspect of your chemistry as it affects your sleep.

## SLEEP HYGIENE

Many of my patients are so tired that they fall asleep throughout the day or feel compelled to take naps. Unfortunately, this interferes with the body's regular circadian rhythm and makes a refreshing nighttime sleep more difficult to achieve, which puts us once again into the downward spirals of insomnia. It is well documented that careful attention to the details that surround sleeping practices, which we call sleep hygiene, will often make a big difference in improving the sleep experience. See Healthy Sleeping Practices for tips on good sleep hygiene.

## Healthy Sleeping Practices

- Don't consume caffeine late in the day.
- Take a hot bath before bed.
- Keep your bedroom dark (any light exposure may interfere with melatonin production).
- Don't consume alcohol near bedtime.
- Keep your bedroom cool.
- If you wake up with acid reflux, try raising the head of the bed one to two inches.
- If you wake up frequently to urinate, consume less fluids in the evening.
- Ignore the clock—paying attention to it is frustrating and not helpful in improving sleep.
- Eat a light snack of high-protein, low-carbohydrate content before bedtime.
- If you wake up with night sweats, check your hormone levels and treat appropriately.
- Go to bed at the same time every night, whether you are tired or not. Consistency in sleep hygiene habits is very important; conversely, inconsistency makes restorative sleep more difficult to achieve.

## SLEEP APNEA AND UPPER AIRWAY RESISTANCE SYNDROME (UARS)

The development of sleep laboratories has shown us that a large segment of our population is prone to sleep apnea or upper airway resistance syndrome (UARS). Sleep apnea is not rare; it is estimated that 20 million Americans have it to some degree! It has been speculated that our dietary changes over the past one hundred years have caused a weakening of our jaw structure, allowing the lower jaw, or mandible, to recede. This in turn results in a dropping back of our tongue into the back of our throat when we sleep, causing sleep apnea or UARS for many people.

Dr. Steven Park, in his brilliant book *Sleep Interrupted,* has demonstrated with clarity how these physiological changes lead directly to sleep apnea and UARS and may be contributing to the rising epidemics of:

- insomnia
- headaches
- high blood pressure and low blood pressure
- diabetes
- obesity
- depression
- heart disease
- erectile dysfunction
- heart attack
- GERD (gastroesophageal reflux disease)
- stroke
- LPRD (laryngopharyngeal reflux disease: chronic throat clearing)
- chronic sinusitis
- chronic postnasal drip
- asthma
- IBS (irritable bowel syndrome)
- anxiety
- ADHD
- MCS (multiple chemical sensitivity)

The basic concept here is that during the deep stages of sleep, and especially REM sleep, all of the muscles of the body relax (except the diaphragm, which is essential for breathing). Since all humans are susceptible to the tongue collapsing to various degrees as a result of this relaxation, different people will obstruct more than others, and many of them will demonstrate this by snoring, sometimes dramatically. Most of us will automatically adjust to this, as best we can, by changing our sleep position from being on our back (the position in which we can obstruct the most easily) to being on our side. Even this positional change may not be sufficient to completely avoid some degree of obstruction.

When obstruction is severe, breathing may stop for many seconds at a time, resulting in a brief loss of oxygen to all of our tissues, which we call apnea. Our need for oxygen is so vital that this condition forces us to wake up, at least a little, so we can take deep breaths again. Laboratory sleep studies have enabled us to measure these awakenings. If breathing stops for more than ten seconds at a time, and there are more than fifteen of these events every hour (called the apnea hypopnea index [AHI]), this is considered the official definition of sleep apnea. If we include patients' symptoms and reduce our criteria to five events every hour, it is estimated that 24 percent of men and 9 percent of women meet these criteria. Clearly sleep apnea is far more common than is usually appreciated and needs to be taken into consideration when we are looking at the components of chronic illness.

When we add to this discussion the newly described condition called UARS, many more individuals will fit into this paradigm. UARS reflects a slight variation on this process, in which when the tongue falls back slightly during sleep, due to increased airflow, a greater vacuum effect is created. That vacuum essentially sucks up acid from the stomach, like a straw, irritating all of the tissues at the back of the throat, extending at times up into the sinus areas. The blockage here may not result in any appreciable snoring, but it can and does result in multiple arousals during sleep, preventing deep, restorative sleep from being maintained. Individuals with UARS often have cold hands, dizziness, lightheadedness, low blood pressure, insomnia, headaches, TMJ, depression, GERD, hypothyroidism, and asthma. These are very common symptoms and conditions, and until recently we had no idea that some of them were related simply to sleep issues.

It is essential, therefore, that we look for sleep apnea and UARS in people with chronic illness, as this is a treatable component. The gold standard for diagnosis is a complete polysomnography study in a sleep laboratory. I am happy to relate that a new technology from the Watermark Medical Company allows us to do a fairly complete sleep study at home for far less money. This technology allows for a panel of electrodes and a nasal prong to be strapped on, just before bedtime, and all of your vital sleep data is recorded while you sleep. The entire setup is contained within a Velcro band that fits gently around the head. The chip of information recorded by the electrodes can be electronically sent to sleep specialists for a detailed reading, allowing us to make these diagnoses with accuracy without having to go through the elaborate process that a hospital-based sleep laboratory requires. I believe this will revolutionize our ability to provide this important information at low cost (about 10 percent of that of a conventional sleep lab).

With this clear diagnosis, we then have several approaches to treatment. The most well-known treatment is called *continuous positive airway pressure* or CPAP, in which the individual is fitted with a mask or nasal device that keeps a gentle, positive pressure on the back of the throat to keep it open all night long. While quite effective, many people are so uncomfortable with the mask and breathing equipment that they cannot tolerate it and discontinue treatment within a few months of beginning it, despite valiant efforts to make it work. Since one of the main causative problems is that of the tongue dropping back into the throat, many dentists can create personally fitted dental appliances that can be worn at night that push the tongue gently forward, improving breathing considerably. Yet another less invasive approach is that of properly fitting a pillow so that an individual's neck position is less likely to allow the tongue to drop back, and we work closely with the Oxygen Pillow Company to provide this alternative service as well.

## RESTLESS LEG SYNDROME (RLS)

A common complaint in many people with chronic fatigue syndrome and fibromyalgia is that of restless leg syndrome (RLS). Part of the difficulty in making this diagnosis is that the full description of this symptom is characteristically vague. Individuals are usually unable to find words that would help us understand exactly what they mean—and that is exactly how they help us to make the diagnosis. They report this vague sense of being unable to lie down comfortably without an intense desire to move their legs, and in fact, often they have to get up and walk about for a while until they can again lie down to try to rest.

As with many of the other conditions described in this book, we saw only a few patients with this diagnosis during the early 1980s, but it is now extremely common. I believe it is yet another manifestation of the global neurological irritability that we are seeing with chronic fatigue syndrome, fibromyalgia, Lyme disease, and other chronic infections. In fact, RLS often resolves when we treat those conditions, making it clear that they are, indeed, related. I have found that the best treatment for this is the use of small doses of Klonopin (0.25 mg to 0.5 mg) at bedtime, to improve sleep while we work on the underlying problem.

I hope that you are persuaded that restorative sleep is vital to the healing process and that we need to examine it carefully as part of our complete healing program.

## FURTHER READING

Park, Stephen Y. *Sleep Interrupted: A Physician Reveals the #1 Reason Why so Many of Us Are Sick and Tired.* New York: Jodev Press, 2008.

Visit Dr. Jacob Teitelbaum's very informative website, www.endfatigue.com, for more on sleep difficulties, sleep supplements, and medications.

Visit www.watermarkmedical.com for more information on Watermark's diagnostic sleep apnea devices as well as a list of providers.

For more information about the Oxygen Pillow, visit info@sleepworks.com or www.O2pillow.com, or contact European Sleep Works directly at 2966 Adeline Street, Berkeley, CA, 94703, (510) 841-5340.

# CHAPTER 21

# Alternative Approaches to Treating Cancer and Autoimmune Diseases

## Dr. Livingston, I Presume?

**D**espite billions of research dollars and the efforts of countless dedicated scientists, we have made only a small amount of progress in the treatment of cancer. In fact, even with newer and more sophisticated diagnostic equipment, the incidence of many cancers continues to increase at an alarming rate. How can this occur? The answer, I suspect, is that our understanding of how the body develops cancer is inadequate. Thus, we must return to a recurring mantra of this book: Without a clear grasp of the cause(s), how can we possibly refine the treatments?

### CONVENTIONAL TREATMENTS OF CANCER

The current conventional treatment of cancer involves three major components: surgery, chemotherapy, and radiation. In fact, in certain states there are actually laws that limit all treatments to those options alone. These treatments certainly have their place, and many forms of cancer are eradicated by their proper use. But first we must try to understand the causes.

We do know something about the factors that allow a body to develop cancer. One of these factors is our genetic structure: We carry certain genes that, if activated, interfere with the proper workings of our immune system. Let me emphasize the phrase "if activated." This means that even if you have inherited genes that may contribute to the creation of cancer, they may never come into play. There is credible evidence that proper diet and lifestyle can prevent this activation from happening.

The healthy functionality of our immune system is the key to preventing and treating cancer. We have an elaborate surveillance system in which special cells within our body are constantly looking for anything foreign, anything that is "not us." If these special cells find abnormal cells that do not perfectly resemble the cell lines with which they are familiar, they either destroy them on the spot or they call for reinforcements to do the job. Sometimes they mistakenly identify our normal cells as being something foreign, to be attacked, and when that happens we are attacking ourselves—which we call autoimmunity. This will be discussed in more detail later in this chapter.

It is generally believed that we constantly generate abnormal, cancerous cells within our bodies, and that our immune system normally identifies and destroys those cells rapidly. When that process breaks down or gets compromised, cancer develops. By definition, a growing cancer means that our immune system has not been able to deal with these abnormal cells properly.

At this point, in conventional medicine, we treat the growing cancer first by surgically excising it, if that is technically possible. Depending on the exact nature of the tumor, we may decide that surgery alone is sufficient treatment, or that additional treatment in the form of chemotherapy or radiation is necessary to eradicate the tumor. Keep in mind that there are many types of cancer, which are usually named after the cell-line and organ from which they grow, and each type is biologically different from the next.

But here's where it can get a little dicey. Both chemotherapy and radiation are destructive treatments that are capable of both destroying the cancer *and* damaging the immune system. I view them as double-edged swords—while they may be lifesaving, they may also interfere with the functions of the immune system that ultimately are necessary for healing. Making the decision to accept chemotherapy or radiation can therefore be quite difficult, and it requires an intimate knowledge about not only the biology of the specific cancer in question, but also the strength of the individual's immune system at that moment in time.

Basically, treating cancer is in some ways similar to treating an infection. While most people believe that infections are cured by the antibiotics they take, this is not really true. The antibiotic, if properly pre-scribed (keeping in mind that we don't have treatment available for most viral infections), will indeed kill off a large number of microor-ganisms, but not all of them. It is our immune system that must come into play to finish the job or mop up. The same is true for treating can-cer: If we can lower the number of abnormal cells in our body using surgery, radiation, or chemotherapy, then we can increase the likelihood that our immune system will be able to get on top of the situation and finish the job of killing these abnormal cells. But if in the process of treatment we have damaged the key system needed for healing, how are we to heal? That is the tricky part, and you can begin to see how difficult it can be for physicians and patients to make these decisions.

Having said all this, please do not lose sight of the fact that this dis-cussion has not begun to include the concept of the cause(s) of cancer, without which more specific treatment cannot be delivered. I believe that this is the major weakness in our approach to cancer today. We spend billions of dollars to refine our surgical procedures and to develop more effective radiation approaches and new chemotherapy drugs. This is well and good, but it doesn't move us any closer to getting to the cause, and without that information, I suspect we cannot make the kind of progress necessary to really make significant inroads to the cure of this disease.

Worse, the industry that cancer treatment has become actually resists the influx of new ideas by invoking the time-honored tradition of claim-ing they are "unproven" and hence potentially dangerous. While I am not advocating the indiscriminate use of unorthodox treatments, the history of cancer treatment is filled with exciting possibilities that were never given even a hint of a true test by the established medical author-ities, and this is to the great detriment of the public.

As entire books have been devoted to this subject, I do not intend to bring all of these treatments to your attention in this one chapter. I would like, however, to discuss one specific approach with which I am quite familiar, and to outline several of the better documented treat-ments. Once again, my goal here is to provide hope that even if you've been told that nothing else can be done, there may indeed be quite a lot that can still be done. I want to point you in that direction.

## THE LIVINGSTON VACCINES

I had the privilege to be the medical director of the Livingston Foundation Medical Center in San Diego from 1991 to 1995. It was there that I learned firsthand of the remarkable research and treatment created by Dr. Virginia Livingston. The story of my experiences at this facility will serve as an excellent example of what I am trying to convey about understanding the cause of cancer.

In 1947, Dr. Virginia Livingston (then Virginia Wuerthele Caspe) held the position of a school physician in New Jersey. While working there, she examined a nurse who had been diagnosed as having Raynaud's disease, a vascular condition in which the fingertips change color and become numb in response to cold temperatures. Livingston found ulcerations on the tips of several fingers, hypersensitivity along the nerves of the patient's arms and legs, and a perforation of the nasal septum, which surprisingly looked a lot like leprosy, a disease with which she was familiar. These findings implied to Dr. Livingston that this nurse actually had scleroderma, an autoimmune disease that often expresses itself as a severe form of Raynaud's syndrome, and this diagnosis was subsequently confirmed by biopsy. Intrigued by the similarities of the patient's symptoms to leprosy, Dr. Livingston made smears from the base of the woman's fingertip ulcers and nasal areas, and then stained them with an acid-fast dye commonly used to diagnose tuberculosis, a bacterium in the same family as leprosy. To Livingston's surprise, and that of her colleagues, the acid-fast stained cells were positive for this family of microorganisms. She treated the nurse with antibiotics known to kill these bacteria, and she recovered completely.

Intrigued by these unusual findings, Dr. Livingston took her work one step further: she grew cultures of these bacteria and injected them into chicks and guinea pigs. Most of the animals became diseased; almost all of the chicks died, and the guinea pigs developed hard areas of their skin similar to what we would find in scleroderma. Some of these areas appeared cancerous, which was quite curious since the incidence of cancer in guinea pigs is very low (1 in 500,000 animals). This suggested to Livingston that scleroderma might actually be caused by these bacteria and might represent a type of slow-growing cancer. She began to screen her cancer patients with this same cell-staining technique and found similar microorganisms in the blood smears of most of them.

Livingston published her initial findings in 1947, and those findings were later confirmed by several researchers at the Pasteur Institute in Brussels, and again by Alan Cantwell, M.D., a dermatologist in Los Angeles who published several papers in reputable journals showing the same results. Other researchers became excited about this work, and several prominent scientists joined Livingston in publishing a series of papers demonstrating the presence of these bacteria in cancer patients. As she and her colleagues investigated further, they realized that these bacteria had pleomorphic properties (meaning that they could change shape and appearance), and they were named *Progenitor cryptocides,* which is Greek for "the hidden killer." In 1949, Dr. Livingston was named head of the new Rutgers-Presbyterian Hospital Laboratory for the Study of Proliferative Diseases. She received grants from the American Cancer Society, *Reader's Digest,* Charles Pfizer and company, Lederle Laboratories, the Abbott Company, and other foundations. She was ready to begin her research in earnest.

At that time, as well as today, it was generally believed that cancer was caused by a virus and not a bacterium. Over the next ten years, Livingston and her fellow researchers were able to demonstrate clearly (and published supporting data) that virtually every type of animal and human cancer contained the bacteria that were similar in structure to tuberculosis and leprosy. The most striking characteristic of these bacteria was that of pleomorphism (another word for cell-wall-deficient bacteria, which we discussed in Chapter 12): the shape-changing capacities of these organisms presented as viral-like bodies in the tumors, which evolved after several months into larger mycoplasma-like L-forms, and then into bacterial rods and filaments. (Mycoplasma organisms are infective microbes whose size is between that of viruses and bacteria.) Other forms of the bacterium were also noted, including larger cysts and spore forms almost reminiscent in appearance to fungi. This means that under the microscope, these bacteria might demonstrate a completely different appearance at different times and under different conditions, making the bacteria very difficult to categorize. Strains of these bacteria were sent to a number of laboratories for identification, but none could really classify them. They were something unknown and new.

With this exciting new concept that the cause of cancer might be this unusual bacterium, Livingston and her colleagues embarked on an attempt to prove it using the time-honored concept called *Koch's postulates.* This system has been used by medicine for decades to prove that a particular infectious agent causes a particular disease. Koch's postulates are:

1. The microorganism must be present in every case of the disease.

2. It must be possible to culture the microorganism outside the host (i.e., the animal) in some artificial culture medium.

3. The inoculation of this culture into a susceptible animal must produce the disease in question.

4. The microorganism must then be able to be found in the inoculated animals and recultured.

By 1950, Livingston's team was able to demonstrate that the *Progenitor cryptocides* indeed fulfilled these criteria, so they published their findings in the *American Journal of the Medical Sciences,* a prominent publication, to a mixed reception. Some scientists were intrigued with this new information, but others tended to dismiss it out of hand because it was not in alignment with the viral theories that were more popular at the time.

Turning to human cancers, Dr. Livingston found that in breast cancer, positive cultures for this bacterium could be directly grown from the blood and lymph glands of cancer patients as well as the tumors themselves. She began to feel that cancer was not simply a localized disease, confined to a single area of the patient's body, but rather a systemic, generalized disease.

As the research proceeded, Livingston became aware of a study that had preceded hers by many years. Similar work had apparently been done by George Clark, a pathologist who in 1920 reported on his successful culturing of a bacterium known as *Glover's cancer organism.* He injected this bacterium into animals, which resulted in the presence of metastasizing tumors. Livingston took this several steps further: she developed a vaccine against the *Progenitor cryptocides* bacterium and demonstrated that she could *protect* animals from getting cancer, even after they were infected by this bacterium, as long they had previously received her vaccine.

Eleanor Alexander-Jackson, a noted expert in tuberculosis and a coinvestigator with Dr. Livingston in her research work, developed breast cancer in 1951. Eleanor underwent radical mastectomy surgery, but then elected to take the vaccine Livingston's team had developed from the *Progenitor cryptocides* bacterium as her follow-up treatment. The other options presented to her were more extensive surgery, cobalt radiation, or chemotherapy, all of which were urged. But Eleanor decided to go with the vaccine instead. She remained cancer free for more than thirty years following the use of this experimental vaccine.

However, the vaccine remained only a research tool until 1965, when a close friend of Livingston pleaded with her to help her husband. The man was diagnosed as having a large lymphoma involving the thymus gland, and he was told it was inoperable because it had already grown into the surrounding tissues. His physicians held out little hope for him. While reluctant, Dr. Livingston agreed to provide him with the vaccine. The patient responded with a complete remission of his cancer and no recurrence over twenty additional years of follow-up.

This seminal event sparked the opening of the Livingston Foundation Medical Center, founded in San Diego, California. Although Dr. Livingston died in 1990, her work continued at the clinic until several years ago, when the clinic was disbanded. However, her vaccines and other treatment materials are still available today from Dr. Edwin McClelland at the San Diego Immunotherapy Clinic, which is unfortunately the only clinic still providing this treatment.

The reason I've taken the time to relate this story is because it details the availability of solid medical research and proven therapeutic results that are still not a part of conventional thinking or treatment. In a 1990 paper published by P. B. Macomber, he asserts that:

> Only a small number of cancer researchers today believe that bacteria play an essential role in the cancer process. Over the years, those few workers who have carried out research supporting this

concept have generally been ignored or discredited. As a result, virtually no discussion of their work can be found in any modern textbook of oncology. Yet collectively, their research indicates that cell wall deficient bacteria are probably constantly associated with animal and human cancers, that these bacteria appear capable of inducing cancer in animals and that immunity to these bacteria sometimes protects experimental animals against certain forms of cancer.

This is what makes this information so exciting: Here we have a safe, nontoxic material, a vaccine made from materials taken from a person's own body, that appears to actually address one of the causes of cancer by stimulating the immune system to improve its own ability to keep this bacterium in check. Isn't this a less drastic solution than chemotherapy or radiation?

At this point you are probably wondering whether the vaccine really worked—it did. Having worked in this clinic for over four years with hundreds of patients with cancer and autoimmune disease, I can attest to its effectiveness. Like any treatment, it worked best if used earlier in the course of the disease. If we could catch patients with breast cancer or colon cancer or brain malignancies early on, we had a superb treatment response. If patients came to us when they were at death's doorstep, we didn't do very well. But even then, we were able to cure or markedly improve from 15 to 20 percent of those individuals, all of whom had already been told by their physicians, "There's nothing more we can do for you." Once again, here was hope, slim at times, but still hope that healing or recovery was still possible.

You don't need to take my word for the effectiveness of this treatment. In 1992, *The New England Journal of Medicine* published a study in which Dr. Barrie Cassileth at the University of Pennsylvania Medical School, who had heard of Dr. Livingston's work and wished to investigate further, compared treatments given at that institution (consisting essentially of conventional approaches) with those provided at the Livingston Clinic. Cassileth demonstrated that both approaches provided *equal* benefits to patients in terms of improvement and cures, but that the Livingston approach was far better tolerated by the patients and had fewer side effects.

## INGRID'S STORY

Ingrid was a sixty-year-old woman from a small town just outside of Springfield, Missouri, who came to see me at the Livingston Clinic for follow-up. She had been diagnosed as having metastatic ovarian cancer several years before, and after several rounds of chemotherapy, following surgery, she was still not well. Ingrid still had residual implants, which are nests of cancer cells that attach to the wall of the peritoneum and the lining of the abdominal and pelvic cavity. She had read about Dr. Livingston's work and made the trip out to San Diego to receive the vaccines as well as the other immune-building materials and diet, along with large doses of intravenous vitamin C. After a two-week course of treatment and instruction, she went home with these materials and continued to use them for several years. When I saw her at the clinic, she was healthy but still not cured, as testing still showed the presence of cancerous ovarian cells.

I continued to treat Ingrid for several years in San Diego, and as luck would have it, I relocated my medical practice to Springfield, Missouri, where I continued to treat her for the next ten years. During that time she did quite well, except for her experiences with several courses of chemotherapy that reduced her white blood cell count to the point that she became susceptible to pneumonia and had several life-threatening bouts with infection, until her immune system could regroup. With the use of the Livingston program and materials, although she was never cured, Ingrid kept her advanced cancer at bay for almost fifteen years! During most of that time, she was able to live a healthy, productive life with her family and community. Her gynecological oncologist, who followed her throughout that period, was initially opposed to her treatment at the Livingston Clinic, but over time he was won over to its benefits. After several years he would reiterate to her the litany that we hear so often in this field: "I don't really understand what you are doing, but please keep it up. It's working." He often commented to her that his conventional treatment was clearly not responsible for her continued excellent state of health and her immune system's ability to keep the metastatic cancer at bay.

Ingrid's story is an excellent example of how an alternative approach, when combined with conventional treatment, produced many years of healthy living.

## OTHER ALTERNATIVE APPROACHES TO CANCER THERAPY

Are there other unique approaches that may be helpful for people with cancer? Yes, actually, too many to include here. While this is not intended to be a comprehensive discussion of the subject, I would like to briefly give a summary of some of those treatments that have the best track records and have been studied in the most detail. There are some general principles of alternative cancer therapy that many alternative clinics incorporate into their programs.

### Diet

There is a great deal of well-documented research showing that certain foods are good for our immune system, and other foods may be detrimental. The major points of agreement include the need to avoid sugar, preservatives, pesticides, and chemicals (translation: eat organic products, especially fresh fruits and vegetables and avoid processed foods). Certain foods, such as broccoli, cauliflower, Brussels sprouts, and kale, contain phytonutrients, which have recently been shown to dramatically improve immune-system functioning. Newer information about the preparation of broccoli, for example, demonstrates that steaming them for one to two minutes is ideal for preserving the nutrients we wish to utilize. Dr. Patrick Quillin, who for many years has served as the nutritional director for Cancer Clinics of America, has written several excellent books on this subject. (See Further Reading.)

### Supplementation

The use of specific nutrients and supplements to improve the immune system is another component to most of these alternative cancer treatment programs. This component includes high doses (25 to 50 g or 25,000 to 50,000 mg) of vitamin C given intravenously, along with selenium, zinc, vitamin A, coenzyme Q10, and other antioxidants. You might wonder why the intravenous route of vitamin C is so essential, but there is significant disagreement about how much vitamin C the body can absorb when given orally. Several studies show that only 100 mg of vitamin C can be absorbed by the body when it is taken as often as every four hours, but others studies done by Dr. Linus Pauling, the winner of two Nobel Prizes, show that much more can be absorbed. The bottom line is that regardless of how much vitamin C can be absorbed when it is taken orally, the intravenous use of vitamin C allows us to provide much more of that nutrient than we could ever get orally. Recent research by Dr. Mark Levine at the National Institutes of Health has finally demonstrated how this works: The high doses of vitamin C given intravenously are converted in the extracellular tissues into high concentrations of hydrogen peroxide, which can then attack the cancer cells.

## Visualization Techniques

Originally proposed and researched by Drs. Carl and Stephanie Simonton, whose work was done at the Cancer Counseling and Research Center at the University of Texas Science Center in San Antonio, Texas, and expanded by others, including Dr. Bernie Siegel, visualization techniques are another major component of most of these programs. Our knowledge of the tongue-twisting field of psychoneuroimmunology shows a clear relationship between our thoughts and feelings and the functioning of our immune system. Carl Simonton was a radiation oncologist who was able to prove that those patients who could picture, or imagine, their immune systems killing off their cancers, did far better clinically than those who did not make use of that faculty. Dozens of subsequent research papers have confirmed that observation. So, a positive outlook coupled with consistent visualization efforts aimed at visually improving the function of the immune system leads to much better outcomes. It is safe, costs nothing but a little time, and has no side effects. Dr. Livingston's program incorporated all of these elements into its treatments.

## Other Remedies

Other programs and concepts for consideration:

- **The Gerson Program.** Named after a pioneering physician who first used high doses of vitamin C intravenously with extensive juicing, coffee enemas, and thyroid supplementation, among other interventions.

- **Macrobiotic Diets.** As popularized by Michio Kushi, uses a fairly austere dietary program to mobilize immune system function.

- **Herbal Treatments.** The Hoxsey treatment, mistletoe (Iscador).

- **Essiac Tea, Pau D'arco, and Mushroom Extracts.** These have been used by thousands of people with considerable success.

- **The Burzynski Antineoplastons.** Dr. Burzynski isolated some unique peptides over thirty years ago and has effectively used them in the treatment of a variety of cancers at his clinic in Houston, Texas.

- **The Immuno-Augmentative Therapy Program (IAP).** Introduced by Lawrence Burton in the Bahamas, IAP also uses some unique peptides in cancer treatment.

- **Biologically Guided Chemotherapy.** Introduced by Emanuel Revici, this therapy utilizes a unique lipid chemistry approach to treatment.

- **Laetrile.** The so-called vitamin B17 had some great success in the 1970s until the product was dramatically diluted by its manufacturer.

- **Homeopathic Approaches.** These include the Sanum remedies and Dr. Vincent Speckhart's electrodermal screening remedies. Dr. Speckhart is an oncologist at the Cancer Cure Foundation in Norfolk, Virginia, who pioneered the use of homeopathics in the treatment of cancer.

These are but a few of the options available to those who are seeking other methods for healing. Several references at the end of this chapter can point you in these directions.

## ALTERNATIVE APPROACHES TO AUTOIMMUNE DISEASES

With other autoimmune diseases, too, the conventional approach is essentially suppressive but does not address the causes of autoimmunity. Autoimmune diseases include rheumatoid arthritis, lupus erythematosus, Hashimoto's thyroiditis, multiple sclerosis, inflammatory bowel disease, and a host of other conditions, many of them less familiar to you. What brings about all of these conditions is an immune system that has become confused—it has started to attack its owner's tissue, mistakenly thinking it is attacking a foreign invader. For example, in rheumatoid arthritis, the immune system attacks the synovium, which is the membrane that lines the joints. When the synovium becomes inflamed, joint pain ensues, and that underlying inflammatory process may become generalized and affect other body tissues. In Hashimoto's thyroiditis, the thyroid gland is attacked, and eventually this process destroys all or part of the thyroid gland, creating a condition of hypothyroidism. In multiple sclerosis, it is the nerve tissue that is inflamed, causing a wide variety of nerve-related symptoms depending on the exact location of the affected tissues and involving, at times, the brain, spinal cord, or peripheral nerves.

For many years, our main therapy for these diseases was (and remains) high-dose cortisone in the form of prednisone. This may, in fact, be lifesaving and absolutely necessary for many patients. However, long-term use of prednisone is associated with a host of serious side effects and ultimately will rarely cure the patient, as it does not address the cause of the problem. There are many newer effective treatments, but they still put the patient at risk for life-threatening infections because they work by suppressing the immune system as a whole, not in a specific way.

On the other hand, there are a host of less toxic approaches that have had success with treating autoimmune diseases. We still do not adequately understand the causes of these conditions; hence, treatments are limited by our lack of knowledge. By looking at this wide variety of treatments, however, we may get a glimpse into what may underlie some of these diseases.

First I would like to refer back to our discussion of the Livingston vaccine. I described the original work that Dr. Livingston did on scleroderma, noting that the same bacterium that caused cancer also appeared to be involved in the development of autoimmune diseases. When she applied her vaccines to those conditions, she had a great deal of success.

I was able to go back into the files and come up with eighteen patients with scleroderma whom we had treated over a number of years. In fact, quite a few of the cases were still active, so I was still following most of them. All were well documented diagnostically from university centers, so the diagnosis was not in question. Of the eighteen we treated with the Livingston vaccine, six were cured, six were markedly improved, and six showed no improvement—that is, two-thirds of the patients responded positively to this treatment! You may not realize it, but conventional medicine is not capable of achieving these results. There is definite benefit with the use of these vaccines in autoimmune illness, and, when it works, it is clearly addressing the cause of that disease in that patient.

Recall also when I described in Chapter 1 the use of hypnosis and emotional release work in curing patients with rheumatoid arthritis and other autoimmune diseases: somehow, this process has the capacity to restore the immune system back into balance.

When we discussed mercury toxicity, I mentioned that this is often associated with autoimmune illness. I have personally seen several cases of rheumatoid arthritis and multiple sclerosis respond beautifully to the removal of mercury, and others have described this as well. What role does heavy metal toxicity play, therefore, in the weakening of the immune system and pushing it toward self-reactivity? Perhaps a very significant one.

We have also commented on the role of food allergy in autoimmunity. Many people with rheumatoid arthritis and inflammatory bowel disease have responded well to or have even been cured by discovering the offending foods and removing them.

Perhaps in a similar way, by restoring balance to the bowel and removing toxins from the system, the practices of fasting, high colonics, and saunas have been used by naturopathic physicians for decades in the service of the successful treatment of these conditions.

More unusual treatments include bee venom therapy. Using controlled bee stings, or bee venom in different forms, has resulted in improvement in people, particularly those with multiple sclerosis and rheumatoid arthritis. While some of you may be shaking your head at this one (I did, too, when I first encountered it), I have seen it work. The venom can be injected just under the skin (subcutaneously) over acupuncture points or into areas of pain, particularly around joints, with great benefit.

Certain infections have been implicated in the development of autoimmunity, especially the HHV6 virus and EBV virus, which we discussed earlier. Improvements have been noted, particularly in multiple sclerosis, by treatments directed at improving the immune system's ability to deal with those viruses, notably with the use of transfer factors.

Again, suggesting the possible involvement of bacterial infection in causing these diseases, Dr. Thomas McPherson Brown from Virginia has published many papers showing the success of using low, long-term doses of tetracyclines (an antibiotic) in treating rheumatoid arthritis. I have personally seen similar results.

We have recently realized that vitamin D is deficient in the majority of our patients, and especially in those with autoimmune disease. By measuring and treating this deficiency, we are seeing great improvements in these patients as well.

Although the following alternative approach sounds so far-fetched as to be dismissed out-of-hand (please don't, since the research on this is extremely well documented), there is a growing understanding that we can use a helminth, or pork whipworm (*Trichuris suis*) orally to effectively treat the intestinal autoimmune problems of Crohn's disease and ulcerative colitis. Joel Weinstock, M.D., Director of the Division of Gastroenterology and Hepatology, Center for Digestive Diseases at the University of Iowa has presented extensively on this subject and it is worth reviewing.

## Low-Dose Allergen (LDA) Therapy

Since the allergy portion of our immune system plays a significant role in many of the conditions we have discussed, an introduction to low dose allergen (LDA) therapy could have been offered when we discussed food allergy or multiple chemical sensitivities. I will include it here in our discussion of autoimmunity.

LDA is a modified version of enzyme-potentiated desensitization (EPD), which was developed in England about forty years ago. It has been pioneered in this country by William (Butch) Shrader, M.D., from Albuquerque, New Mexico, and taught to physicians through the American Academy of Environmental Medicine. It consists of injections administered every two months initially just under the skin of the forearm. It utilizes very tiny amounts of a wide array of allergens, directed against inhalants, chemicals, mold, and food irritants. These solutions are given with a unique enzyme mixture that improves the immunizing effects. The results of these injections are to stimulate T-regulatory cells in such a way that they are prompted to "forget" what they are allergic to. Unlike other allergy treatments, LDA often results in a complete cure of the allergy and does not require lifelong injections for benefits to be appreciated.

In the context of this chapter, specific ingredients in the injections have been shown to help reverse inflammatory bowel disease and every form of autoimmune illness. We have seen patients with severe IBS recover completely with a series of these injections. As a general rule, it is harder to treat multiple chemical sensitivities (MCS), where the allergic process appears to have gotten more deeply imbedded into the immune system. Here is an example of how well this procedure may work.

## LARRY'S STORY

Larry was a forty-year-old university professor who presented to us two years ago with severe multiple chemical sensitivities. His problems began in 1999 following blood clots to his legs and lungs and continued with another pulmonary embolus in 2006. After his hospital stay that year, he became highly sensitive to many foods and spices that he had eaten all his life without any difficulties. By January 2007, he realized that he had become highly reactive to all kinds of chemicals and odors, which he correctly termed "volatile organic compounds," and received the official diagnosis of MCS.

He found that even brief exposures to some of these chemicals caused reactions so severe that he would be confined to bed for days at a time with overwhelming fatigue, anxiety, depression and brain fog. His teaching was limited now, because an hour's exposure in the classroom to undergraduates, many of whom wore the chemicals he could not tolerate, would incapacitate him for long periods of time. He was frightened that he would lose his job and his career, and that he would get even worse. He wrote: "I lived by trial and error, learning what I could tolerate without getting totally sick and continued that way."

He first saw me in September 2010, and we started him on DHEA and vitamin D based on measured deficiencies. A stool culture showed several pathogenic bacteria and Candida, and we treated those as well. In December 2010 we began LDA and we have now completed ten rounds of treatment. Although still sensitive, he is able to go into the classroom and teach with only minor setbacks afterward. His energy is markedly improved, his mind is clear, and he feels like he has gotten his life back. We later added the methylation protocol and some homeopathic treatments, which have augmented the entire program.

As a general rule, once an individual starts developing chemical sensitivities, they become more and more reactive over time, until they are barely able to leave their home.

Larry has continued to progress with treatments to the point that he is no longer limited, and we are hopeful that with the next series of injections with LDA, he will recover completely.

---

Once you begin to investigate these alternative treatment areas more deeply, you will find many other options for treatment that are worthy of exploration. Hope abounds. Sometimes you have to take a creative step back to get a better perspective on the whole situation. This may help you to realize that no, you really haven't tried everything available in your search for a cure.

## FURTHER READING

Brown, Thomas McPherson, et al., Relationship Between Mycoplasma Antibodies and Rheumatoid Factors, *Arthritis and Rheumatism,* Vol. 19, pp. 649–650 (1976).

Cassileth, Barrie, et al. "Survival and quality of life among patients receiving unproven as compared with conventional cancer therapy." *The New England Journal of Medicine* 324, no. 17 (1991): 1180–1185.

Diamond, W. J., and Cowden, W. L. *Alternative Medicine Definitive Guide to Cancer.* Tiburon, CA: Future Medicine Publishing, 1997.

Elliott, D. E. and Weinstock, J. V., "Helminthic therapy: using worms to treat immune-mediated diseases." *Advances in Experimental Medicine and Biology* 666 (2009): 157–166.

Gonzalez-Rey, Elena and Delgado, Mario. "Vasoactive intestinal peptide and regulatory T-cell induction: a new mechanism and therapeutic potential for immune homeostasis." *Trends in Molecular Medicine* 13(2007): 241–251.

Livingston, Virginia. *Conquest of Cancer: Vaccines and Diet.* New York: Franklin Watts, 1983.

Macomber, P. B. "Cancer and Cell Wall Deficient Bacteria." *Medical Hypotheses* 32 (1990): 1–9.

Quillin, Patrick. *Beating Cancer with Nutrition.* 4th ed. Carlsbad, CA: Nutrition Times Press, 2005.

Summers, RW, Elliott, DE, Urban, JF, Thompson, R, and Weinstock, JV, Trichuris suis Therapy In Crohn's Disease *Gut,* Vol 54, pp. 87–90, (2005).

*Unconventional Cancer Treatments.* Washington: U.S. Congress Office of Technology Assessment, 1990.

# CHAPTER 22

# The Growing Epidemic of Autism

## How It All Fits Together

I've enjoyed creating mildly amusing subchapter titles for this book, but somehow it doesn't feel right to do that with a chapter on autism. Having a good sense of humor is one thing, but there is absolutely nothing amusing about having a child who is struggling to function in every way.

When I went to medical school at the University of Chicago, I had some contact with Dr. Bruno Bettelheim, the medical researcher who had his Autogenic School at the University. He was one of the first physicians to try to come up with a strategy to help these challenged children. Back then, autism was extremely rare and mostly thought to be due to unusual genetic imbalances. Curing or improving autism in those days was always felt to be a minor miracle.

Today, we are in the midst of an epidemic of autism. One in eighty children is now diagnosed with autism, and in certain communities that incidence has increased to one in fifty. It is also important to realize that the presentation or form of this disease has changed considerably. Previously, children diagnosed with autism were clearly "abnormal" from the very start of their lives. They never developed properly or walked or talked, or made meaningful contact with their caregivers. What we are *now* seeing is different, and shows up primarily as *regressive* autism. What this means is that these children are the product of normal births, grow and develop normally, talk and walk and cuddle, and connect well to their parents and family up until a certain moment in time, usually between six months and two years of age, when they take a sudden and dramatic backward turn and *lose* those abilities, hence the word "regressive." Unfortunately, the conventional medical understanding and approach to autism is to place these children on multiple, powerful psychotropic medications in order to control their symptoms of out-of-control behaviors, tantrums, tics, "stimming" activities (repetitive body movements), and withdrawal from social contact.

As with many of the concepts presented in this book, "controlling" or "managing" symptoms can never result in cure, as these treatments do not begin to address the cause. Most conventional physicians do not believe we have adequate knowledge of the cause, and hence they do not make any efforts to work with it. And once again, it is *my* belief, shared with an increasing number of physicians, that we have, indeed, learned a great deal about this new and epidemic form of autism, and that we can treat it by getting closer to the causes.

With autism we have a very fascinating story. The search for a cause began with Dr. Bernard Rimland's vision that a new approach to this illness was desperately needed. In 1967 he founded the Autism Research Institute, which started by involving the parents of these children by asking them to rate the benefits of all of the treatments their children were receiving. The process was simple: Parents scored each treatment as better, worse, or unchanged for every intervention they tried, including both conventional and alternative approaches. Over the course of time, thousands of parents heard about, and became a part of this process so that a significant number of observations accumulated. Using a scale of one as meaning "unchanged," less than one as meaning "worse," and more than one as "better," it was clear that most medications were, if anything, mildly helpful. But a host of natural treatments clearly made much bigger positive differences. It was noted that dietary changes that affect digestion, including removing milk and wheat from the diet and looking for food allergies, made big differences and were highly rated by parents. In addition, by treating occult intestinal yeast and bacterial infections; removing toxins from the body, especially mercury and lead; treating methylation defects; and supplementing with specific vitamins and nutrients, children showed a marked improvement. It became clear that each child was unique and had to be approached individually for progress to be made. Using this approach, some children were cured and most got better. Does this whole process sound familiar? It should, since I've devoted whole chapters of this book to all of these interventions and concepts.

To put this together into a more cohesive picture, what I believe we are seeing is that the same biochemical imbalances and stressors (heavy metal toxicity, food allergy, chronic candidiasis, and methylation chemistry dysfunction) will affect individuals at different ages, or different stages of development, in different ways. So, for example, mercury toxicity in an infant with a rapidly developing nervous system will have a different presentation, with different symptoms (such as autism spectrum or ADHD) than a thirty-year-old (such as fatigue or joint pain), than an elderly person (such as cognitive impairment, Parkinson's disease, or dementia). I believe that understanding this concept ties together what otherwise appears to be very disparate chronic illnesses.

Looking at this bigger picture, more and more researchers became intrigued with the possibility of helping these children. Some of the most passionate, of course, began their journey when their own children were diagnosed with autism. When your own child is affected, this is powerful motivation to find answers. In 1995, this body of information evolved into the Defeat Autism Now! movement, which continues to integrate new information and research into the treatment program, and is taught to more and more physicians as time moves on. As parents learned about the epidemic, their need to have these treatments available and supervised by knowledgeable physicians led to this whole biomedical approach, and large medical conferences are held several times a year to facilitate this exchange of information.

What we have learned thus far is that the key areas of imbalance in these children are their brain chemistry (no surprise) and their intestines. The latter shouldn't be much of a surprise, either, to readers of this book, when we remember that the gut contains more neurotransmitters than the brain and is often referred to as the "second brain." The gut is also associated with the immune system, 60 percent of which is present in the gut as the gut-associated lymphoid tissue (GALT), which we discussed in Chapter 8. Although the neurological effects of autism are in many ways more obvious, the intestinal symptoms have long been present but mostly overlooked. During recent autism conferences, gastroenterologist after gastroenterologist has presented material on the marked prevalence of every type of intestinal diagnosis in autistic children. The autism groups have discovered that treating this condition starts with "normalizing" gut function.

The key imbalances in intestinal physiology, which we've seen in other chronic conditions, are food allergies, especially sensitivity to casein (milk protein) and gluten (wheat protein) and to soy products. One major starting point for treatment is to take autistic children off of each of these, separately—followed, if necessary with more elaborate tests for other food allergies. If an autistic child improves with this simple elimination diet, we're off to a good start. Typically we begin with the removal of all milk products for up to three weeks, and watch the child for their symptomatic response. Usually children who are sensitive to milk products will start to improve in the first week. Then, for up to three months (although again, I usually see improvement in those who are going to respond to this intervention in the first week), we remove all wheat products. It is common for us to need to remove soy products as well for a more complete evaluation, since there is a 25 percent crossover allergic reaction between milk and soy. Approximately 70 percent of children with regressive autism will benefit from this intervention (see Chapter 7).

Next, we turn our attention to evaluating for intestinal dysbiosis, particularly looking for the presence of the yeast *Candida* or toxic bacteria. I would personally estimate that up to 80 percent of the children that I treat respond well to this treatment. Please see Chapter 8 for a more thorough discussion of this important subject.

Then we shift our attention to the evaluation of toxicities: heavy metal toxicity (especially mercury and lead), which we reviewed in Chapters 10 and 19, and chemicals and pesticide exposure to our affected children, which we discuss in Chapter 23. New studies show a clear relationship between exposure to pesticides in agricultural settings and the incidence of autism.

Studies also suggest a relationship between vaccine usage and autism in several ways. First, until recently, many childhood vaccines contained significant amounts of thimerosol, a mercury-containing preservative. When vaccines were "bundled," meaning multiple vaccines were administrated to children all at the same time, doctors were inadvertently injecting large amounts of mercury into these children's systems. While this situation has improved somewhat, thimerosol is still present in appreciable amounts in the flu vaccine, which is now recommended for most children, and in smaller amounts in other vaccines. Second, and separately, there is reason to suspect that the measles component of the MMR vaccine, which is administered as a live virus vaccine, may actually cause infection in some cases. Although the virus in the vaccine is supposed to be "attenuated" or weakened, and therefore benign, it would appear that this may not always be so, and the ensuing infection may trigger the onset of autism in susceptible children. *Susceptible* is the operative word here.

We have gathered enough information that a new model to understand and treat autism has been proposed by the Autism Research Institute group. That model includes our discussion about food sensitivities, chronic intestinal yeast infection, and multiple toxic exposures. We have begun to learn more about the details of genetic predisposition, which we can now measure by simple blood tests of single nucleotide peptides (SNPs), which are genetic mutations that can pinpoint more precisely where biochemical imbalance is likely to occur. This offers us a clear starting point for treating these imbalances. Dr. Amy Yasko has pioneered our understanding of some of these key areas in the arena of disordered methylation chemistry (see Chapter 14). Additionally, a wide variety of nutritional supplements have been shown to improve these biochemical and genetic predispositions.

We have also noted that many of these autistic children have received multiple rounds of antibiotics for a wide variety of infections, and for some children, this may have triggered the excessive growth of yeast and toxic bacteria in their intestines, which in turn may aggravate or lead to food allergies or sensitivities.

In the complex interweaving of these interconnected components of illness, we can begin to see how each piece of this puzzle affects the next piece, and the next. We therefore have to look at as much of the entire picture that we can find, and treat all of it. This means that if we miss an important piece—for example, mercury toxicity—we may not be able to adequately treat methylation imbalances, as minuscule amounts of mercury can profoundly affect the body's ability to methylate. In turn, by its depletion of glutathione (because of poor methylation chemistry), the body is not able to adequately detoxify other environmental exposures and/or deal appropriately with vaccine exposures and/or pesticide and chemical exposures (some of which have yet to be defined). The bottom line is that these challenged children cannot produce the natural materials that they require for healing.

Jill James at the University of Arkansas has recently completed some meticulous research that provides clear evidence for the presence of these methylation deficiencies and also demonstrates excellent clinical response to a simple supplement-replacement treatment program. She is currently engaged in a more extensive research effort to both study and treat these imbalances

As heartbreaking as the diagnosis of autism is for all parents, our new awareness of all the components that may be factors in autism provides real hope for parents and children and gives us impetus to embrace new models of understanding and treatment.

## ISAAC'S STORY

Isaac was a five-year-old boy who I initially saw in May 2007 at his mother's request. He had seen two medical specialists who had made the diagnosis of Asperger's syndrome, which is currently considered a variety of autism. Isaac had developed completely normally up until about two years of age, when his behavior began to change. His mother felt that these changes seemed to occur following vaccinations he received at that time. His mother observed that Isaac would often go into his own little world. He was having increasing difficulty making contact with others, especially if they were not family or well known to him. When people would get too close, Isaac would literally tell them to back off, or he would shy away. It was difficult to get him to leave the house without taking a host of toys with him to keep him entertained. He appeared to be quite intelligent (common with Asperger's children), but his speech was "off" at times, and he was not yet toilet trained.

When we tested his stool, he had overgrowth of the yeast Candida albicans as well as the toxic bacteria Klebsiella and Enterobacter. We initially treated him with Nystatin and Diflucan, and prescribed the use of melatonin for difficulties with sleep, which is commonly seen in autistic children. The use of the methylation protocol made a big difference in Isaac's behaviors from the moment we started, although initially there was a slight increase in his tic behaviors and some social withdrawal. As he was a big milk drinker, we eliminated the consumption of milk to see if this would help. It made little difference.

He was placed in a special educational program at school, and within a few months of beginning our treatment, he was completely potty trained and was able to ride the bus to school by himself. At this point his mother felt he was 40 percent better than when we'd started. When we retested his stool in March 2008, he had several bacterial pathogens and two species of Candida on culture. At that time he'd gone off the methylation protocol and was encouraged to resume it, which he did. We treated the intestinal overgrowth with Nizoral uva ursi (a herb with antibacterial properties), and undecylenic acid (an antifungal), and he improved markedly. By the end of summer school in July 2008, he was ready to resume regular classes with just a small amount of time out of his school day (twenty-five minutes) devoted to special training in speech and motor skills. He was able to interact much better with his peers and no longer exhibited the anxiety and tics he had prior to treatment. His mother was thrilled with his progress.

Unfortunately, just prior to the start of school, Isaac was given four "bundled" immunizations, including the MMR vaccine. His mother had been concerned about his possible reactions to the immunizations, but Isaac's pediatrician had been insistent. Within twenty-four hours of the shots, his mother reported that "I've never seen him so nervous or jumpy." Over that first week his regression continued as he became increasingly fearful and began holding back his willingness to interact with others. One week after the immunizations he broke out in a finely grained, red rash all over his body. We were moving back to square one.

Fortunately, with resumption of his supplements and a little time, this exacerbation resolved within a few weeks and Isaac resumed school activities successfully; his gains in behavioral function returned, and he has continued to make steady progress.

## NINA'S STORY

In January 2008, I had my first visit with a very delightful seven-year-old named Nina. She had been diagnosed with petit mal ("absence") seizures at the age of three, and over time had been found to have difficulties with focus and attention and sleep. She was closely followed by a pediatric neurologist who diagnosed her with ADHD (which some experts consider part of the autism spectrum). He placed her on the medication Concerta, which seemed to help initially. After eighteen months, her mother had begun to wonder whether the side effects of Concerta were outweighing its benefits. Nina had also been placed on Lamictal an antiseizure medication, but EEGs (brain wave testing) continued to be abnormal, and she had frequent headaches, averaging three times a week. The family did quite a bit of research over the Internet, as is common among my patients, and they were hoping that some of these newer concepts could be helpful for their young girl.

At our first visit, after collecting the appropriate information, I began with some osteopathic cranial manipulation. When Nina returned, six weeks later, her headaches were markedly diminished. We added vitamin B6 and the supplement L-taurine to her program. We started the process of looking for food allergies and possible heavy metal toxicity. On a DMPS challenge test, small amounts of nickel, lead, and mercury toxicity were discovered, and she was started on DMSA twice weekly. One mg of melatonin was added at bedtime.

By Nina's next visit, her sleep had improved, headaches were rare, and she had experienced only one significant seizure. Her mother told me that Nina was substantially better already. We added the methylation supplement protocol and continued her cranial manipulation. By July her mother reported to us that Nina was "happier and more energetic." She was no longer having any seizure activity, and headaches were few and far between. She had been tutored that summer and had caught up to her grade level for educational instruction. Her mother was able to say that her concentration and focus had improved dramatically. Off medication completely, she no longer exhibited symptoms of ADHD and was free from seizures.

---

You can see how combining a nutritional approach with osteopathic manipulation, removing toxins, and providing methylation support was able to produce marked improvement for Nina in just six months. Restoring health and improved brain function for these children is clearly possible. I am delighted to report that I have personally successfully treated dozens of these children who have been returned to complete health.

I am in awe of the effort and dedication of the parents of these autistic children. Their willingness to step out of conventional boundaries to find the help their children need is inspiring. Many will not accept "you'll just have to learn to live with this" as an answer, and through their efforts, we are pushed to dig ever deeper for answers and solutions. The good news is that this intense search is often rewarded with the evolution of a healthier, happier child, and a grateful family.

## FURTHER READING

McCandless, Jacquelyn. *Children with Starving Brains: A Medical Treatment Guide for Autism Spectrum Disorder.* Putney, VT: Bramble Books, 2007. Dr. McCandless's book provides an excellent overview of the concepts and treatments available for autism.

McCarthy, Jenny. *Louder Than Words: A Mother's Journey in Healing Autism.* New York: Dutton, 2007.

Pangborn, Jon and Sidney Baker. *Autism: Effective Biomedical Treatments: Individuality in an Epidemic* (with 2007 Supplement available). San Diego, CA: Autism Research Institute, 2005. This book, along with a great deal more information, is available from www.AutismResearchInstitute.com.

For a more in-depth discussion of autism, I gave a two-hour presentation to the Mendocino Coast District Hospital, which was filmed for public television, and I invite the reader to visit the website: www.mcdh.org and go to Health & Wellness, then go to Video on Demand for this free presentation.

# PART FIVE

# The Bigger Picture
## A Look Toward the
## Future

---

With all of this new information about alternative health treatments that I've shared with you here, I would like to complete this book by putting it all into perspective. Thus far, much of this book has been directed to the evolving understanding of how body chemistry becomes disordered and can be repaired, so that we can better understand and treat chronic illness. We have also explored ways in which we can improve our anatomical knowledge and treatment of chronic pain.

Now I'd like to step back a little and look at the bigger picture.

The first area for us to explore is an important one: Why have so many individuals become ill in such a short period of time? Despite all of the advances of modern medicine, why are cancer and autoimmune diseases and fibromyalgia and chronic fatigue and autism and Alzheimer's disease becoming more prevalent and at an alarming rate? Many scientists have studied this critical question, and to many of us it appears that what has changed is our environment. Chapter 23 explores how this has happened and attempts to clarify this frightening phenomenon.

Next I will explore the importance of listening. This includes the need for me to listen really carefully to what my patients are expressing, so that I can begin the diagnostic process. It also includes the patient's need to listen to the messages provided to them by their own bodies so that they can take action accordingly. Chapter 24 delves into this vital but often overlooked area.

Chapter 25 is an unusual one in that it highlights the seldom discussed relationship between money and healing. It looks at the important interactions between patients and healthcare providers as decisions are made about how to spend money in the service of health.

Chapter 26 will explore the spiritual dimensions of health and healing. Our attitudes toward our illness, our bodies, and our families play an important role in determining how we will fare healthwise. We must courageously explore this to prevent anything from limiting the natural healing processes.

In the Afterword I will present a brief story about the power of caring.

CHAPTER 23

# Ecotoxicity: How the Environment Is Making You Sick

## Only the Tip of the Iceberg

Having gotten this far in the book, the most obvious question you may be asking yourself is, "Why is all of this biochemical mayhem happening now?" There must be reasons for the emergence of these epidemics of fibromyalgia, chronic fatigue, autism, ADHD, asthma, cancer, Alzheimer's disease, and Parkinson's disease. I believe there are, but none are scientifically confirmed or proven to date. Despite the lack of proof, I can't help but speculate on what might be going on here. I, and many other physicians and scientists, suspect that there are chemical, energetic, emotional, and spiritual components involved.

### OUR TOXIC RELATIONSHIP WITH TECHNOLOGY

For starters, we seem to have lost touch with what makes us human. As a species relatively new to this planet, we seem to think we can create a world separate from the one we are actually living in. For most of our time on earth, we have lived in some degree of harmony with nature: we hunted, we farmed, we gathered, we fished. We have always had to pay careful attention to the natural world so that we could survive and thrive. If we hunted- or fished-out a species of game, we had to leave that area and move on, so we learned not to do so. If we didn't treat the soil properly, we learned that it would not produce in abundance.

But now, we have rather suddenly lost our intimate contact with the natural world. The most glaring example of this is the insidious proliferation of technology in our lives. You can't go anywhere without being deluged by media. It is a rare restaurant that doesn't have multiple television sets visible, or even audible, from every seat in the room. When, and how, did that happen? Airports are filled with people on cell phones, talking in raised voices, seemingly oblivious to the world around them. This forces all of those in their vicinity (in this instance, me) to respond in some way to this outpouring of sound energy. I can try to tune it out, become irritated, listen in with interest, or wear blocking earphones to deal with it. But deal with it I must, because I can't just ignore it. Perversely, this distances me from my own perceptions and my own life and intrudes upon my physiology in a most insidious, unhealthy way. And everyone takes it for granted to the point that they are oblivious to what is happening around them.

I take a walk with my family in a natural setting, and almost every jogger, bicyclist, or fellow walker is wearing earphones and plugged in to a virtual world that separates them from the world they're walking in. I see this as a deeply spiritual problem. For many of us, one of the simplest ways to be close to God (whatever that concept means to us) is through a natural setting: a sunrise, or sunset, or blue sky with fleecy clouds, or a stream running through a grove of trees, or a field of flowers. But if we're not present to it—because we are "living" in a virtual reality—even if we are walking through this natural world, we no longer take the time to see, hear, smell, or feel it—our real world. So we have the bizarre experience of being in it, but not really taking part in it. And as this strange dissociation from the world we inhabit continues, we have an increasingly strained relationship with the natural world. We're seeing now the effects of global warming, cutting down the rain forests, of building huge tracts of housing on good farmland, of eating genetically modified foods, of using untested chemicals in abundance on our soils and in our homes and schools. No one seems to be paying much attention to the bigger picture. It may seem that I am exaggerating or overstating the case here, but without trying to be an alarmist, I am deeply concerned for the universe that we are creating and for the effects this toxic universe will have on our children and grandchildren.

We become numb. So numb that our media has to resort to gorier pictures and more intense fear-based news and images to get our attention. So numb that even the most realistic movies barely move our audiences. I read studies that show that an extraordinary percentage of Americans are currently taking antidepressants, and from a glance at my patient population, I believe them. Basically, antidepressants numb us. So how, in this numb, stressed, out-of-touch universe that we are creating, can we even notice how we feel? It's simple—we can't. Our bodies were designed to notice imbalances and bring them to our attention so that we could fix them. If we can't do that, because we're numb, we can get really sick before we realize we need to do something about it. When we do come to our senses, we often find our medical providers have no idea how to address these profound biological imbalances in any sort of practical way. So they tell us we are stressed and it's "in our heads." And what will they give us for treatment? Why, more antidepressants of course!

Where else can we go for help? Where must we look in order to address this problem?

We have to go *home*. And by home I mean back into our own bodies, our own lives—to recover ourselves. It's not outside of us; it's inside. And we've lost the awareness of both what we need to do and how to do it. That means we need to change our relationship with technology. I am not suggesting that technology is malevolent or that it has no place in our modern world. I am saying that for many of us our relationship to it is way out of balance, and most important, we need to be *aware* of that relationship so that we don't completely lose contact with the natural world. But how can we do that? Many people I have known work in front of computer screens all day long and come home to more of the same—the Internet. We pay bills with it, buy airline tickets with it, "surf" it, communicate with it, are beguiled by it. It's not just going to go away, nor should it.

We clearly need a new relationship with technology. How exactly can we do this? I am not going to propose glib answers to a very difficult problem, but I can say that the essence of this problem lies with the loss of our abilities to notice our own thoughts, our own feelings, our own perceptions—because we are deluged with electronic stimuli all around us. We must find some personal way to slow the deluge for long enough that we can recover ourselves and not allow ourselves to be swept up into it. I believe we can, and must, do this.

A recent breakthrough in understanding this relationship and doing something about it comes from the publication of the book *Earthing* by Clinton Ober and colleagues. They clarify the direct relationship of the earth to our bodies by demonstrating that the surface of the earth is teeming with negative electrons, which are capable of quenching the buildup of free radicals in our bodies that produce inflammation—if we can just make contact with them. They have shown that if we can go barefoot, in direct contact with the ground, for thirty to forty minutes daily, it can have a profound effect on pain, sleep, cognition, immune function, and hormonal function. For those who cannot go barefoot in their environment, they have created special sheets, mattresses, and pads that connect to the grounded outlets in our homes, so that we can sleep grounded—or "earthed"—and restore our health using this simple, safe, nondrug process.

## PESTICIDES AND CHEMICALS

Another major need for awareness is found in these classic words:

> For the first time in the history of the world, every human being is now subjected to contact with dangerous chemicals, from the moment of conception until death. In the less than two decades of their use, the synthetic pesticides have been so thoroughly distributed throughout the animate and inanimate world that they occur virtually everywhere. . . . To adjust to these chemicals would require time on the scale that is nature's; it would require not merely the years of a man's life but the life of generations.

It may come as a shock to learn that these are not newly penned sentences, but were written in 1962 by Rachel Carson in her groundbreaking book, *Silent Spring.* The "two decades" she refers to are now six. Although the publishing of her book led to the prohibition of the pesticide DDT, a recent study showed that even forty years after DDT was banned from our environment, fat biopsies (most chemicals are stored in our fat cells) performed just a few years ago show that virtually all of us still have DDT in our bodies!

The chemical industry releases approximately 500 new chemicals every year. It is estimated that there are perhaps 80,000 chemicals in our environment, and only 500 of them have been adequately studied in terms of their effects upon humans! What is worse, there are virtually no studies of how those chemicals interact with each other. We are swimming in a sea of chemicals that are almost certainly poisoning our bodies, our whole world, and we are not allowing ourselves to measure the profound effects that this has upon us. This should be a terrifying fact, but most of us go along blithely with the attitude that "if they were dangerous, surely we'd know by now." But remember, it took many years for us to discover that DDT had profound effects on the environment and our hormones and needed to be banned. It took years to "prove" that cigarettes were dangerous to our health, and yet the consumption of cigarettes continues (especially in our youth) at an alarming rate. We pride ourselves on our education and what we have learned, yet we often do not act on that knowledge in a healthy way.

We have evidence that many plastics and common chemicals in our environment are xenoestrogens, *xeno* signifying "foreign." What this means is that these unnatural chemicals are so close in their biochemical structure to our natural hormones (estrogen being the one named here) that they behave like hormones in our bodies, not only confusing our chemistry, but making it nearly impossible to eliminate or detoxify them because they are not natural. We have discovered that many of these chemicals, even in exquisitely small amounts, block and interfere with our normal hormonal function. There is solid evidence that male sperm counts and fertility rates, globally, have decreased by more than 50 percent in the past twenty years! Do we not think this is really significant? No, we gloss over it, hoping, like the epidemics of disease that we are currently seeing, that magically it will all just go away. We rarely drink the water available to us from our taps anymore. We drink from plastic bottles, thinking that this water is purer—but is it? We have reasons to doubt. What *is* safe? I no longer know the answer to that question, but I do know that we must find out, and soon.

I, and many others, believe that it is our polluted world that is making us so sick. Some of us are more sensitive than others, and those are the ones who are coming into my office now. I don't think it will be very long before these numbers increase dramatically. Those who have felt immune to these exposures will have to deal with these environmental toxins, too. This means *polluted* not only in terms of chemicals, but also pollutions of noise, electromagnetic radiation, information, and stressors, among others. This is sensory stimulation overload, with which we are ill equipped to cope, yet we rarely even acknowledge it.

For example, as I write these words on my word processor, I am aware that after about two hours in front of this screen, I can no longer think clearly. Unless I allow my awareness of this to become conscious, I will continue to plug along until I can no longer write coherently. If I can then go outside or take a walk, this "fogginess" will fade after thirty minutes to an hour. Discussions with hundreds of patients over the past few years have convinced me that my experience is not unique. Where is cyberspace, actually?

Some of my patients are much more sensitive to electromagnetic effects and are rendered almost nonfunctional with everyday exposures. The proliferation of radio towers and beacons in our world has gone almost unnoticed, but that does not mean that they do not affect us. When I worked with the neurosurgeon Dr. Norman Shealy, from Fair Grove, Missouri, a dozen years ago, by carefully monitoring the brain waves of sensitive patients, we were able to clearly demonstrate that in the presence of electromagnetic radiation (a simple electric clock, for example, placed near their heads), those patients would move from functional alpha and beta brain-wave patterns into random delta brain-wave patterns that correlated precisely with their loss of cognitive function. Dr. Shealy termed this *electromagnetic dysthymia,* which I believe is an excellent name for this medical condition.

In the past six months, I have had three patients present to me with extreme electromagnetic sensitivity, which began as soon as Smart Meters were installed by Pacific Gas and Electric into their homes in northern California. I suspect that this, too, is the tip of the iceberg.

I believe that we will be seeing new and even more unusual illnesses emerge out of this toxicity. An example of this is Morgellons disease, an unexplained systemic condition with strange skin effects. People with this newly recognized illness (which has been linked to Lyme disease) vividly describe the emergence of what appears to be threads from lesions of their skin. These threads have been described as clear, blue, or red, and have been dismissed by many practitioners as a delusional observation by those individuals. At the November 2012 annual ILADS meeting, researchers from Stanford were able to demonstrate that these "threads" are actually filaments of keratin (the protein that makes up our hair and nails) and that the blue color represents fragments of reduced hemoglobin. Doesn't this sound frightening? It would be hard to imagine developing this illness and not being emotionally upset by its manifestations.

Until now, most people have taken an "I'm okay, so what's *your* problem?" approach to hearing of these experiences. The implication here is that an innate sensitivity to chemicals, electromagnetic radiation, or foods must be somehow psychological rather than a physical, non-controllable reaction. When viewed with a little more compassion, one might say instead, "There but for the grace of God go I." Neither of these attitudes reflect a realistic compassion or understanding of the problem. Sorry, but we're all in this together as an integral part of this universe. There is no rug to sweep this under. It will not go away.

The Japanese nuclear disaster of Fukushima released (and is still releasing) untold amounts of radiation into our environment. The informational ban imposed by our government ten days after the event scares me more than whatever actual knowledge we might have about those radioactive isotopes. I live on the West Coast of this nation, and I believe, as a physician, I need to know what my patients are being exposed to, if I am to help them. But that information is not available to me. Is that not of concern?

It is like there is an elephant in the room, and we have all agreed not to notice it or talk about it. Remember our discussion on cognitive dissonance? Here is another example. You see, the elephant *is* in the room and denying its existence will not make it go away. There are obviously tremendous economic pressures to avoid this discussion, but I am convinced that our lives will depend on our immediate admission of this huge problem and not delaying one more minute to deal with it. I don't see that we have any choice.

If we're going to talk about health, we have to include the bigger picture in this discussion, and I hope that this chapter will get you thinking about it.

## *FURTHER READING*

Carson, Rachel. *Silent Spring*. New York: Houghton Mifflin Company, 1962. Quotations from page 7 and page 15.

Colborn, Theo, Dianne Dumanoski, and John Peterson Myers. *Our Stolen Future*. New York: Plume Books, 1997.

Krimsky, Sheldon. *Hormonal Chaos: The Scientific and Social Origins of the Environmental Endocrine Hypothesis*. Baltimore, MD: Johns Hopkins University Press, 2000.

Ober, Clinton, Stephen T. Sinatra, and Martin Zucker. *Earthing*. Laguna Beach, CA: Basic Health Publications, 2010.

# CHAPTER 24

# Deep Listening: Understanding the Human Side of Complex Chronic Illness

## Friends, Americans, Countrymen: Lend Me Your Ears

I t is difficult for me to explain to others the process we use to help people regain their health. I think the reason for this is, in essence, that it is too simple and does not fit into the model used in standard medical practice today. That model, as we've discussed, includes a very brief interview with the patient followed by lots of high-tech testing and prescription writing. It seems pretty obvious that this model has no real chance of working or being effective, since it eliminates the possibility of allowing the patients to tell their story and express their feelings—there's simply no time for real healing.

In my opinion, helping people boils down to intense listening and remaining ever attentive to patients' descriptions of their personal health. While listening to patients should obviously be the most important part of a physician's medical interaction, I throw in the word *intense* to emphasize that this does not mean merely sitting in the same room with my patients but reflects the hard work of really paying attention to them as they speak. This means listening to not only their words but to the pauses between words, to the words that are emphasized (hence more emotionally charged and meaningful), as well as observing their body language and facial expressions as they relate their stories—looking for things such as leaning forward in the chair, legs abruptly crossed, sudden deep breaths, sighing, and eye contact or lack thereof. In short, I must take in the totality of that individual human being and allow the totality of my being to get involved, so that it registers information about what is really important to that individual. Somewhere in that presentation are the clues I need to be of help. If, as occurs more and more frequently as electronic medical records become commonplace, the physician is busy working at her computer with her back to the patient, keying in the patient's information, or if she is pressed for time and wondering how she can possibly fit everything into the morning schedule—including her required "output of productivity"—it is clear that meaningful listening cannot take place. Somewhere in the past fifteen to twenty years, we went from being physicians to becoming *providers,* and that seemingly simple linguistic change has had a profound impact on the practice of medicine.

The closest model that approximates a process of deep listening may be found in the field of osteopathic medicine, which we discussed in Chapter 17. This may come as a surprise to some who aren't aware of the osteopathic profession or how it differs from that of conventional medicine. There is, in fact, a deep philosophical underpinning to osteopathy, which is surprisingly absent from that of allopathic medicine. There are four basic principles of osteopathy, as outlined by the renowned doctor of osteopathy Rollin Becker in his book *Life in Motion:*

1. The body is a unit.

2. The body possesses self-regulatory mechanisms.

3. Structure and function are reciprocally interrelated.

4. Rational therapy is based upon an understanding of the body's self-regulatory mechanism and the body's interrelationship of structure and function.

Based on those principles are the following steps that Dr. Becker recommends to address healing the body:

1. Accept the "living mechanism" in you and the patient. The "mechanism" is an osteopathic term that refers to the natural, inherent motion in all body tissues and "feeling the mechanism" is a phrase which describes the effort made by a physician to place one's hands on a patient's body and sit quietly to perceive those motions.

2. Life is always trying to express health and we need to be in tune with that expression to correctly assist our patient in their healing process.

3. Surrender comes after acceptance. Accept the fact that what the mechanism is telling you is true.

4. Develop palpatory skills. The body is smarter than you are, so learn to learn from it.

A great deal of wisdom is buried in these succinct comments. What Dr. Becker is driving at is this: that at the heart of our interaction with our patients, we need to change our thinking that our job is to fix what is wrong with the patient. Rather, we must find a way to understand that there is a deep core of health in these patients already manifest— after all, here they are in front of you, fully alive. This understanding needs to be accessed by both doctor and patient in order to harness the forces of healing. The key word here is *accessed*. This means listening, sensing, feeling, and paying attention, so that we can reach the patient's own self-healing mechanisms and begin to move forward.

The beauty and brilliance of this concept is that it recognizes that patients essentially heal themselves; we don't do the healing for them. Missing the truth of this is what has gotten the field of medicine moving down the wrong path in its approach to evaluating and treating chronic illness. In the current philosophy of conventional medicine, both physicians and patients are under the misperception that the physician is doing the healing. So the patient turns over the responsibility for healing to the physician, and the physician accepts it. If both accept this unwritten contract, they are in trouble. The patients are abnegating their own responsibilities here, and the doctor is taking on responsibilities that are literally impossible to fulfill. This is a recipe for disaster.

Let's take a simple example. If a patient comes to me with pneumonia, and I give him a prescription for antibiotics, he assumes I've done my job. He thinks the antibiotic prescription will heal him. If he gets better, unfortunately he will assume that I and/or the antibiotic have cured him. But no antibiotic is capable of wiping out every bacterial cell in his body. The antibiotic allows the patient's immune system to get a leg up, a good head start on the process. But the total eradication of the bacterial or viral invaders is completely dependent on the ability of that patient's immune system to finish the job and mop up. If it can't do that, the infection will continue to smolder and the patient will stay sick.

Healing, therefore, depends almost entirely on the patient's own immune system and not on the antibiotic. I suspect that both patients and physicians have forgotten this, which leads to the odd interactions that now occur between them. If the patient isn't getting well after being given an antibiotic, the doctor feels responsible: "Maybe I used the wrong medication, or maybe I didn't prescribe it for long enough, or maybe I've got the wrong diagnosis, or maybe . . ." To make things worse, the patient comes to believe that the doctor is responsible and returns to the physician's office worried and upset. But what's really happened here is that we've missed the point. The doctor and patient need to work together to harness the patient's healing powers and find some way to stimulate that immune system to work properly.

Perhaps the patient I mentioned earlier contracted pneumonia because he was stressed or exhausted from working long hours or dealing with a family emergency. Perhaps the structure of his rib cage and his ability to ventilate properly were compromised by a seemingly insignificant fall—last week, perhaps, when he caught himself awkwardly by grabbing on to a railing as he fell. Perhaps his immune system was weakened by his diet (for several weeks he had consumed almost nothing but fast food eaten on the run). All of this may need to be addressed before true healing can take place. But if both physician and patient believe that a different antibiotic should be prescribed (in the seven minutes allotted to this visit) and that this will fix the problem, there is the distinct possibility that both are likely to be mistaken and that healing will be delayed even more. The patient may then get even more ill and even more frustrated with the lack of progress from this medical interaction.

Returning to the principles of osteopathy expressed by Dr. Becker, from the beginning of our doctor-patient interaction, we should be searching for the sources of health that the patient brings to the table and trying to harness those to move forward. What exactly might this mean? Well, it could mean discussing the patient's current stressors and ways to cope better. It could mean discussing the effects of smoking tobacco and drinking alcohol. It could mean discussing diet and its effect on the immune system: sugar consumption and fast foods are known to weaken the immune system, so if you are treating your pneumonia and eat most of your meals out at fast-food restaurants, this might well influence your ability to heal. It could mean discussing the use of herbs and supplements that are known to improve immune functioning, such as vitamin C, echinacea, goldenseal, or colloidal silver for an acute viral infection. It could mean exploring the patient's physical structure more carefully. Does the patient have any restrictions to movement of their rib cage or diaphragm (caused by an old fall, or tension perennially held in the chest) that could be treated manually and would allow better ventilation of the lungs and speed healing (or prevent recurrence).

Searching for those sources of health could also mean looking at the patient's thinking process and emotional response to pneumonia: "I always get sick every winter, and it goes to my lungs and it takes months to go away" is a common expression. This predisposes that individual to get sick because he believes he *will* get sick every winter, which opens the door to the very event he fears by direct effects of his beliefs and thoughts upon the immune system. The mind exerts a powerful effect on the body that is not always beneficial, unless it is recognized and harnessed properly.

You can see that doing this sort of analysis cannot easily be limited to a seven-minute visit. Clearly, our treatment model not only takes more time, but it also presents a completely different approach to how we provide medical care. This model is more comprehensive, more logical and inclusive, and more likely to produce the desired results. It also changes the relationship or interaction between the doctor and the patient so we are working together to understand the healing process, and we each have a responsibility for the outcome.

This is not a new paradigm. It has been around for centuries and is beautifully expressed in the osteopathic principles quoted earlier.

Unfortunately, the paradigm has been neglected, and we are all the worse for it. The more complicated and long-standing a patient's suffering, the more difficult it is for us to understand it and to find some way to recognize, encourage, and stimulate the patient's own healing abilities to come forth. For some individuals, this information is so deeply buried that this process is going to take a lot of time. However, the clues will only emerge through careful listening and repeated visits to the drawing board.

## CALVIN'S STORY

I had been treating sixty-two-year-old Calvin for several years. Initially he had only needed some osteopathic manipulation for recurrent neck and shoulder pain, and I was able to help him with that over the course of several months. Several years later, he developed the onset of intense chest pain, and we referred him to a cardiologist who was able to diagnose a coronary artery obstruction and treat it properly with stenting.

However, for the past two years Calvin had been complaining of vague muscle aches and cramping, along with the insidious onset of difficulty with focus and concentration and headaches. Since Calvin was an attorney, this was more than a mere nuisance; it was interfering with his work. He had also gotten a bit depressed, which we presumed came from some serious stressors in his life, and we placed him on a small dose of antidepressant medication. After consultation with other physicians, he began to suspect that he had had undiagnosed adult-onset attention-deficit difficulties for many years, and I prescribed Adderall, a stimulant, to help with his mental functioning. The medication appeared to be working, and he basically seemed content with our treatment. But six months later he came into the office with a new complaint: he had developed paresthesias (sensations of numbness and tingling) down both arms and legs, in patterns that did not reflect the usual nerve distributions.

This new symptom produced that "aha" moment, when suddenly information falls into place and makes sense. I asked Calvin about whether he had noticed any mold in his home. I was not surprised when he related that he had smelled a lot of "mustiness" over what appeared to be the open beams of his home, and that there had been some water leakage from his furnace several years ago as well. When his home was carefully inspected, he did indeed have mold over many areas of his home, and most worrisome, in the heating and cooling systems.

We treated the mold toxicity (see Chapter 11) with Questran and Actos, and within two weeks Cal's paresthesias had virtually disappeared, along with the headaches. He reported marked improvement in his muscle spasms and cramps that had bothered him for several years. His depression had lifted, and the focus and concentration issues had significantly improved, so that he no longer required his stimulant or antidepressant medication.

He still needed to proceed with the remediation of his home, and he did have mild to moderate exacerbations of his symptoms each time he was additionally exposed to mold in other settings. But the mystery of his illness had been resolved.

---

This story illustrates how important it is that each practitioner (in this case, myself) continues to keep his mind and ears open so that he can receive new information and process it properly. In this case, not an unusual one, one new symptomatic detail allowed all of the previous data to fall into a clear and understandable pattern. Now we had something to work with, and now we could move toward healing. As I continue to reiterate, without a clear diagnosis, it is awfully difficult to achieve healing. And it is only by listening, carefully and wholeheartedly, that we can obtain the clues we need to make that diagnosis.

## FURTHER READING

Brooks, Rachel, ed. *Life in Motion: The Osteopathic Vision of Rollin E. Becker, D.O.* Portland, OR: Stillness Press, 2001.

Sutherland, Adah S., and Anne Wales, eds. *Contributions of Thought: The Collected Writings of William Garner Sutherland, D.O.* 2nd ed. Fort Worth, TX: Sutherland Cranial Teaching Foundation, Inc., 1998.

## CHAPTER 25

# The Price of Healing

---

## Does It Really Cost an Arm and a Leg?

Now we come to a very difficult subject: the interaction between finances, attitudes, and healing. Sometimes, money does matter. But it's more complicated than that. If you had a severe, debilitating illness that interfered with all aspects of your life, how much would you pay to correct it? From my perspective as a physician with his sights set on healing (since this is the world I inhabit every day), everyone should be willing to move heaven and earth to regain their health. As biased as my perspective is, I still believe that few things are more important than your health. However, I have also learned that health, or healing, is not everyone else's highest goal or value. So I have to modify my goals—after all, it is your healthcare visit—so that they align with those of my patients.

People will endlessly surprise me. Some of my wealthier patients will not spend a dime more than their insurance coverage will allow on their health. They will not authorize testing or use supplements or medications, and they will even say, "If my insurance company won't cover it, I must not need it." I am not aware of the enlightened philosophical nature of insurance companies or of their intense desire to be helpful at all times. Rather, my experience is that they will make a serious effort to deny claims whenever possible. On the other hand, many of my less wealthy patients will do everything they can to pay for every test I suggest and take to heart every recommendation I make. Guess which type of patient does the best?

In a way, a person's attitudes toward the costs of medical care are a

Rorschach test, or barometer, of the kind of progress they'll make. Those who tell me from the beginning, "Do what it takes; I just want to get better," almost invariably do so. Those who "nickel and dime" me from the first visit—"Which of those tests are the cheapest? Which ones can I put off?" are likely to have a halting, up-and-down healing process, with excruciatingly slow to little improvement.

While some of this is about money, much more is about attitude. A genuine, wholehearted desire to get well is required for a successful journey. Rarely does healing occur when a patient is not committed to the effort involved. Making dietary changes, taking supplements and medications at the correct times, learning relaxation techniques, really looking into one's attitudes toward healing, or changing the stressful impediments of one's life takes a great deal of effort and discipline. Without that effort, healing may not occur. I don't just sit down and write a prescription or hand you a supplement and then you simply heal. Usually, once chronic illness has set in, quite a bit more effort is necessary.

When the patient does not care to know about the financial aspects of our interactions ("Oh, my insurance will take care of all of this"), or if they have no financial responsibility for that interaction (as with Medicaid or Medicare patients), it profoundly impacts our interaction. Since our current medical system is largely based around these systems, we have lost the awareness of how important understanding the financial aspect of care can be to the healing process. If people are not personally involved in the process of paying for the services they receive, they are distanced from our interaction and this diminishes their responsibility for their part of our interaction. It is not the amount of money that is exchanged that matters. I am simply stating that the actual exchange of money between us, no matter how small, adds immeasurably to our interaction. When it doesn't happen, it may have significant impact on our relationship.

One example of how the exchange of money impacts the healthcare relationship would be how Medicare patients respond to the financial aspects of our relationship. When a patient pays me, directly, for my services, we have an immediate connection. They become a part of their healing. When they don't pay me directly, and the payment comes from "out there, somewhere," they are no longer involved in this process.

For many years, I did not accept "assignment" from Medicare. That simply means that Medicare patients paid me directly, on the day they saw me, and Medicare reimbursed them several weeks later. When we switched to accepting assignment this meant that the patient did not pay me at the time of service, and we were reimbursed later by Medicare. You might think that there was not much difference in those scenarios, but actually there was. When patients paid me on the day of their office visit, they did much better. They were much more committed to their healing and took a more active part in everything we outlined. When they no longer paid me directly, that commitment significantly decreased, and those patients shifted into an "if Medicare doesn't cover it, I must not need it" framework. They were much less likely to take an active part in their own care. They increasingly declined testing or procedures that weren't completely covered by Medicare. Consequently, their progress dropped off significantly.

Please understand that I am well aware that many of my disabled and elderly patients have a limited income and truly have very little extra money to spend on their health care. This adds enormously to their difficulties in getting their health care needs met. Nor do I want to suggest that if they would merely accept every test and treatment that I offer them (no matter how expensive that may be) that I can guarantee that their health will improve spectacularly and their delight will know no bounds. I am merely trying to broach the difficult and complicated subject of the relationship of spending money to achieve healing.

Unfortunately, many useful tests, critical to diagnosis and treatment, which are described throughout this book, are not covered by insurance. Without these tests, we may be working with our hands tied behind our backs. For example, the best tests for Lyme disease (the Igenix Western Blot tests), or measuring the details of methylation chemistry are not covered by insurance. Without an understanding of, and commitment to the cost of medical procedures, we are trying to swim upstream. How willing patients are to shoulder some of these costs is a clear statement of their commitment to healing. Those patients who wrestle with me over the cost of each and every test definitely do not fare as well. Their lack of commitment to healing is readily seen in this arena and reflects predictably on our treatment outcomes. Again, I am deeply aware of how difficult it is for many of my patients to afford the cost of this testing, and I do not want to minimize the often agonizing process of how they must decide their priorities. I simply want to be sure that we factor this into our discussions.

Regarding disability, when a patient presents with a desire for disability, often the patient does not understand that this is antithetical to the healing process. It is not possible to seek both healing and financial gain simultaneously. Psychologically, when a person determines that they are entitled to disability, the vast majority cannot do so in good faith without unconsciously taking on the role of suffering, forever, in order to earn it. Alas, I cannot recall a single patient who was on, or sought, permanent disability who was able to fully heal. Often, as such individuals make progress, they get to the point where they are almost well, and then they invariably have a serious setback that puts us back to square one. It is almost as if psychologically, they cannot give up their disability, even for health. Now, for some, the reason may be financial, fearing loss of income and not knowing if they can return to the workforce, even if they are well. For others, disability represents a sort of entitlement or justification of a life of hard work: "I've worked hard all my life, and now I am hurt, and they owe me." While these may be completely valid and entirely true statement, unfortunately many of these people don't realize that within this context, change or healing is not possible. They may be stuck in a pattern of disability and suffering forever.

This brings up the problems related to Medicaid patients. With even less income, often on survival level, how can those people afford the kinds of tests and treatment that we describe in these pages? For the most part, they can't. This raises all sorts of ethical issues that we wrestle with constantly. How can we help those patients with little or no money? *Can* we help them? I don't have the answers to these questions, but they are important concerns for all of us. It is heartening that groups of dedicated doctors who primarily serve the underprivileged are beginning to come together to explore ways of doing just this. A recent example of this occurred at a medical conference put on by the Bay Area Integrative Medicine for the Underserved physicians in July 2011 in Santa Rosa, California, which brought together experts from all over the country to address these issues. (For more information visit www.IM4Us.org.)

The bottom line here is that each patient needs to search his or her own heart for a true commitment to healing. The more sincere that desire, the more likely that they will reach their goal. No matter how ill a patient is, I believe that healing is possible. I, of course, do not do the healing. That's between God and my patient. But I can help to provide the hope and the blueprint by which healing may be achieved.

# CHAPTER 26

# To Make Things Worse . . . or Better

---

## The Only Thing We Have to Fear Is Fear Itself

Even if you have a severe illness and have been told by experts that "there is nothing that can be done," it is usually possible to find a wide variety of ways to improve your ability to cope with it. No matter what the medical condition may be, we tend to make it worse (often much worse) by how we view it. Our attitude toward the problem profoundly affects our experience with the problem. Whenever we sense that something is wrong, fear enters the picture. Could my illness be really serious? Could I die? Will I suffer? How much will I suffer? How long will it last? Will I be able to keep on working at my job? What will happen to my family? Will I be able to pay the bills? These are unavoidable questions that flood our minds with doubt and fear as soon as we begin to feel poorly. Even a simple cold can begin the process of bringing fear to the table. Understandably, this fear is magnified intensely when the illness we are beginning to come to grips with is cancer, unremitting pain or fatigue, an autoimmune disease with a long medical name, the onset of senility or uncontrollable tremors, shortness of breath, autistic symptoms, or whatever you have that brings these real concerns to mind.

Fear is compounded by our history with those symptoms. If a close relative died of cancer, and it was a difficult death accompanied by some of the awful side effects of radiation or chemotherapy, any symptoms that remind us of this history are all the more terrifying. It is not unusual for me to see a patient who has a very treatable tumor refuse all conventional medical treatment. They are often under the mistaken impression that their tumor is frighteningly similar to that of their loved one who died so miserably. Fear closes our minds to options for treatment and takes on a life of its own, adding significant weight to our medical burden.

This is the added element of suffering. We suffer from our medical condition, and then we *add* to it all of our fear, frustration, anger, irritability, feelings of loss and abandonment (by family and friends and God), hopelessness, and despair. These added feelings are not necessarily based on what is actually happening in this very moment, but on our worries about what might happen, could happen, sometime in the future. Dwelling on the past and on what we used to be able to do before we got sick, or when we used to be healthy, active, or loved, or when life was good, serves very little purpose. Living in the past only pushes us to make comparisons that have no value. Yes, when we were twenty, we were stronger, more physically fit, had more stamina, and perhaps had more hair. That may have been ten, twenty, thirty, or forty years ago. But life has moved along, and hopefully we have moved along with it. To bemoan the past only brings a huge dimension of suffering to our current problems. If we can let go of those comparisons and live in the present, we can eliminate that dimension of suffering we carry with us and truly decrease our current pain and worry. Similarly, if we dwell on our fears about what might happen next, this also adds enormously to our burden of suffering.

A wonderful example of what can happen when you deal with this fear is that of my friend and teacher, Jim Jealous, D.O. Twenty-five years ago, Jim was diagnosed with cancer of the thyroid gland. "There was a hard nodule on the right side [of his thyroid] and every time I touched it I was very frightened," Jim recalled. He felt certain that he could not be healed until he had mastered his fears about what might happen next. So instead of choosing surgery immediately, which is what most people would do, Jim wrestled with his fears for the next year and a half, until he felt that he was no longer controlled by them. At that point, to his surprise, when the thyroid was rebiopsied, the cancer was completely gone and never returned.

Another example is that of Ginny Morgan, a superb teacher of insight meditation. She developed breast cancer and went through the usual treatments of surgery, followed by radiation and chemotherapy.

Her first rounds of treatment were very difficult and accompanied by intense nausea, throwing up, loss of appetite, hair loss, and lots of pain and fatigue. As she applied her knowledge of meditation to her treatment, she recognized how she was adding to the difficulty of her experience by not being aware of how her fear and anger and frustration had become a part of her world. As she learned to let go of those future-based thoughts and ideas ("What will happen to me if . . ."), many of her symptoms decreased and, in fact, disappeared. The cancer had not been completely cured, but her suffering from it had diminished greatly. When it recurred, several years later, and was found to have metastasized to her spine, her oncologist was astonished to discover that she was not in any pain. This was not a magical cure, but was the result of her awareness of how she added to her suffering when she brought the past and the future into the present moment. Years later, although she still had cancer, she remained upbeat and maintained a very active teaching schedule. She spent happy hours with her family and was a living inspiration and demonstration of how the correct attitude toward illness can enrich one's life immeasurably until her death one year ago.

This is a phenomenon that I see every day. To some extent, every person who becomes ill has to struggle with the way in which they may add to their suffering by their own reaction to their illness. Sometimes these attitudes are familial or cultural. When I worked in Minnesota, which has a large Scandinavian population, it was clear that "being strong," a form of stoicism, is a deeply ingrained part of that culture. While it is not true, of course, that everyone of Scandinavian descent feels this way, there was still an intense cultural value that was taught at an early age to not give in to emotional expression because it is seen as a sign of weakness. Under many circumstances, this attitude can be useful. However, if a suffering human being needs to express their emotion in order to release it, and cannot do so because of cultural restraint, this can add to their burden.

Many people are not aware that emotional energy is contained and held directly in our musculoskeletal system. Yes, the memories of our emotions are held in our minds, but the actual experience of emotion, if not released, moves into the weakest areas of our muscles and fascia (the connective tissue wrapping our muscles). What I am saying here is that unreleased emotion remains in our bodies (not in our minds) and adds directly to the burden of pain and suffering we are experiencing. Moreover, it takes physical energy to hold onto those emotions, and this depletes our energy reserves significantly. For those who are already experiencing fatigue as a part of their chronic illness, using energy in this way is a luxury that one may not be able to afford. Unless we understand this principle and allow some form of release to occur, this burden will not simply go away. Time alone cannot cure it.

In clinical practice we can often see the presence of this emotional backlog when we are treating a muscle and there is a sudden release of tension from that muscle. While this is a *physical* release, sometimes, when the muscle finally lets go, an unexpected flow of intense emotion occurs, often accompanied by a memory of when that emotion was first acquired. Massage therapists and acupuncturists see this with some regularity. I have referred to this information in Chapter 17, but it is so important that I think it bears repeating. It helps to understand this phenomena, as otherwise an individual may become afraid or upset by the experience, and may attempt to repress it further by tightening up the muscles that need to be released.

Commonly we see the presence of shaking or trembling accompany this release, and this simply represents the body's need to release the stored tension. If this emotional release, with or without shaking and trembling, is allowed to occur, this can add to the healing experience. But if it is suppressed, it can make the person feel even worse. We all have our own bodily areas where we are predisposed to store this tension, such as the neck and shoulders, stomach, bronchial tubes, and lower back. This stored tension can then be directly related to the onset of headaches, ulcers, asthma, and back pain, and of course, much more.

The key to using this information is to be really honest with yourself about your feelings about your illness. Are you making it worse by allowing yourself to dwell on your worries? Following a long discussion of this subject, one of my patients recently returned to our office, thrilled to discover that her self-pity had played a major part in her symptoms. When she fully acknowledged and owned her self-pity, and turned her worries over to God, her irritable bowel disease and bronchospasm improved almost overnight. A wonderful book on this healing area is Byron Katie's *Loving What Is,* which contains a very clear outline and method of how to analyze these forces in your life.

You can do this. You can search your mind, by praying or meditating or just being quiet, and discover how you are adding to your suffering . . . and let it go. It is extremely important that you do this, because sometimes we can't heal otherwise.

Recently, a young woman came into my practice with another presentation worthy of our discussion. Although she had not yet graduated from college, she had already seen a vast array of healers of all kinds. She had significant pain, constantly, across her neck and shoulders and down her back. She had had extensive physical therapy, massages of every type and description, extensive prolotherapy requiring long, regular plane trips to another city, and repeated x-rays and MRI scans that failed to provide a treatable cause for her pain. After several visits and treatment with osteopathic manipulation, which produced only fleeting benefit, she expressed the desire to be treated much more frequently as perhaps that might help. We squeezed her into our busy schedule, but somehow it was never convenient for her to make those visits and she cancelled them all at the last minute. At that point, I declined to offer her further visits, as I felt she was the youngest *notcher* I had yet encountered. The word *notcher* is my own term for certain patients who, like the gunslingers of the Old West, put a "notch" in their belt for every medical encounter they have. While not common, several times a year a patient will appear in my office with a complex story, and they appear to be much more concerned with *telling* that story than with getting any help with their medical condition.

What distinguished this young woman from other notchers was her age and her arrogance. As she related her story, she clearly couldn't be bothered to recall the names of any of the physicians or health practitioners she had seen. Like other patients who exhibit this odd behavior, eventually it becomes clear that they are more interested in proving that you (and anybody else) can't help them, than they are in making any progress. This response to treatment is so unusual that it took a long time for me to realize the value of this behavior for these patients. Initially, it made no sense to me. Why would anyone continue to suffer and sabotage all efforts at treatment for which they were paying good money? It took a while, but I finally understood that for these unfortunate individuals, this lack of progress demonstrated, once again (another notch on that belt) that no one could help them, reaffirming in their own minds how really special and unique they were. It seems that it was more important for them to be special than to get well. Getting better, for them, was a matter of secondary importance.

When I worked at the Shealy Institute, where Dr. Norman Shealy was quite well known for his advanced ideas in the treatment of pain and depression, we would occasionally receive these visits. At first, I didn't understand what was happening, but after a while it began to make sense. People would arrive from a distant city, and as they presented their history to us, it was filled with long descriptions of all the famous people they'd seen and how unsuccessful that had been. Initially, we would work really hard to help them, only to find that nothing worked. Then, they would trundle off, almost happy, now that once again another famous clinic hadn't been able to help them. By appearing to work with us, and not improving, they were demonstrating to themselves that they were so unique that no one, not even the best clinicians, could help them. After a while, we learned to recognize this behavior early in their presentation by the long but dearly held litany of all the wonderful doctors who had failed to help them. I learned to respond to this by the end of our interview by sadly shaking my head and commiserating with them: Yes, they were unique and special and way too complicated for us to deal with. Paradoxically, they would smile at this and happily wander off, delighted that they could add yet another famous clinic to their resume that proved, beyond doubt, how special they and their illness were.

The underlying thought process here runs something like: "You probably can't help me (after all, no one else has), but I will show up and see what you can do." Showing up is not enough. Unless each person is personally involved in his healing process, I, Neil Nathan, can't cure him. God can, but only if the individual embraces his role in his illness. At best, I am a catalyst or helper, one who enables the patient to access his own healing resources.

It is always a concern, when we think that someone may be a "notcher," that we may be guilty of arrogance ourselves. We must always remain aware that maybe, just maybe, we are missing a rare diagnosis and not doing right by that patient. We must always come to the table with as much humility as we can genuinely muster.

Each patient, must, therefore, search his and her own heart for the deepest truths about their own attitudes toward healing. While sometimes that part of their journey is the most difficult, it may also be the most rewarding. Healing requires not just hope, but also commitment and dedication.

Chodron, Pema. *When Things Fall Apart: Heart Advice for Difficult Times.* Boston: Shambhala Publications, 1997.

Katie, Byron. *Loving What Is.* New York: Three Rivers Press, 2002

Kornfield, Jack. *A Path With Heart.* New York: Bantam Books, 1993.

Sarno, John E. *Healing Back Pain: The Mind-Body Connection.* New York: Warner Books, 1991.

# The Most Valuable Thing
# I've Ever Done

---

When it comes to the emotional and spiritual components of healing, words often cannot adequately communicate what we are feeling.

I'd like to end this book with a story from my early experiences in medical practice. Even now, years later, I look back on this moment as perhaps my finest work, although in reality, I cannot know how this event was perceived by others. I just know how I felt and hopefully, that is sufficient.

In the fall of 1985, while working in private practice in Duluth, Minnesota, I was asked by my colleagues in another clinic to cover for them for just a few hours while they held their annual Labor Day picnic for their clinic staff and families. I readily agreed to provide coverage, but was surprised when a local emergency room called me but a few minutes after they'd signed out to me. An elderly gentleman, a longtime patient of one of my colleagues, had just presented to the emergency room in severe cardiac failure, and they were admitting him to the hospital. I immediately ran over to the hospital, where cardiologists had taken over the intensive care procedures and were trying to revive him and save his life. Unfortunately, his heart attack had been a massive one, and after a valiant attempt at resuscitation this gentleman died.

His wife was sitting anxiously in the waiting area of the intensive care unit, her hands clasped together, a look of great distress upon her face. I was uncertain how to approach her. After all, I did not know her husband, and during his intense resuscitation, I never even had the chance to exchange a few words. How could I comfort her? She did not know me, and I could not honestly provide even a few platitudes about her husband, whom I had not known. I was lost for words. I had no idea what to do. I only knew that she was dreadfully upset and needed comforting.

So I sat down next to her and explained who I was, how I came to be there, and what had happened to her husband. Not knowing what else to do, I took her hand and held it for a moment. There was nothing more to say. She seemed reluctant for me to pull my hand away, so I just sat with her, holding her hand. Time passed, and when I finally patted her hand and stood up to say good-bye, I was astonished that two hours had passed.

Although I had, for all intents and purposes, done almost nothing during those hours, I left the hospital feeling that I had truly been of service that day. I still feel that this may have been the most valuable thing I've ever done in my forty-one years of medical practice.

Sometimes we get caught up in the details of our medical world, and we get wrapped up in all of the technology and the chemistry and the multisyllabic words and difficult-to-pronounce names. And sometimes, life reminds us that we are, essentially, only human, and that it is our caring for others that is our finest gift.

# APPENDIX

## MEDICAL CONDITIONS DISCUSSED IN THE CASE

| CASE HISTORY | CHAPTER | CONDITION(S)/SUBJECT(S) DISCUSSED |
|---|---|---|
| Travis's Story | Chapter 3 | Adrenal (DHEA) deficiency |
| | | Persistent rib cage pain |
| Karen's Story | Chapter 3 | Fibromyalgia/chronic fatigue |
| | | Adrenal (DHEA) deficiency |
| Carla's Story | Chapter 3 | Fibromyalgia/chronic fatigue |
| | | Adrenal deficiency (DHEA, cortisol, mineralocorticoids) |
| Jim's Story | Chapter 4 | Magnesium deficiency |
| Tanya's Story | Chapter 5 | Wilson's syndrome |
| | | Fibromyalgia/chronic fatigue |
| | | Adrenal deficiency (DHEA) |
| Ellie's Story | Chapter 5 | Wilson's syndrome |
| | | Chronic fatigue |
| Estelle's Story | Chapter 5 | Iodine deficiency |
| | | Fibromyalgia/chronic fatigue |
| Kristy's Story | Chapter 6 | Estrogen deficiency |
| | | Fibromyalgia/chronic fatigue |
| | | Adrenal deficiency (DHEA) |
| Sheldon's Story | Chapter 6 | Testosterone deficiency |
| | | Chronic fatigue |
| Clarence's Story | Chapter 7 | Food allergy and joint pain |
| Olivia's Story | Chapter 7 | Food allergy and inflammatory bowel disease (Crohn's) |

| Norma's Story | Chapter 7 | Food allergy and rheumatoid arthritis |
|---|---|---|
| **CASE HISTORY** | **CHAPTER** | **CONDITION(S)/SUBJECT(S) DISCUSSED** |
| Rochelle's Story | Chapter 8 | Dysbiosis and irritable bowel syndrome (IBS) |
| Nick's Story | Chapter 8 | Food allergy and failure to thrive |
| | | Bronchospasm (asthma), eczema |
| Karl's Story | Chapter 9 | Hypoglycemia |
| | | Chronic fatigue and depression |
| Ed's Story | Chapter 10 | Mercury toxicity, chronic fatigue, cognitive dysfunction |
| Patrick's Story | Chapter 10 | Root canal, hypertension, cognitive dysfunction, weakness, shoulder pain |
| Maureen's Story | Chapter 11 | Mold toxicity, severe nausea, mood swings, cognitive dysfunction |
| | | Multiple chemical sensitivities (MCS), headaches |
| Barbara's Story | Chapter 11 | Mold toxicity, seizures, migraines, cognitive dysfunction, numbness and tingling (paresthesias) |
| Mark's Story | Chapter 12 | Chronic Lyme disease |
| | | Headaches, fatigue, cognitive dysfunction |
| Kendra's Story | Chapter 12 | Chronic EBV (Epstein-Barr syndrome) |
| | | Chronic fatigue |
| | | Cognitive dysfunction |
| Hallie's Story | Chapter 12 | Chronic EBV |
| | | Fibromyalgia |
| Katy's Story | Chapter 13 | Amino acid deficiencies |
| | | Fibromyalgia |
| Bernice's Story | Chapter 13 | Amino acid deficiencies |
| | | Parkinson's disease |

| Case History | Chapter | Condition(s)/Subject(s) Discussed |
|---|---|---|
| Edward's Story | Chapter 14 | Methylation chemistry dysfunction |
| | | Chronic fatigue, Wilson's syndrome, cortisol deficiency DHEA deficiency, magnesium deficiency |
| Henry's Story | Chapter 15 | Sciatica from Pyriformis syndrome |
| | | Trigger point therapy |
| Heidi's Story | Chapter 17 | Chronic facial pain |
| | | Craniosacral manipulation |
| Kristina's Story | Chapter 18 | Chronic low back (sacroiliac) pain |
| | | Migraine headaches |
| | | Osteopathic and craniosacral |
| manipulation | | |
| | | Prolotherapy |
| My Story | Chapter 18 | Prolotherapy, chronic shoulder pain |
| Betty's Story | Chapter 18 | Prolotherapy, chronic knee pain |
| Kitty's Story | Chapter 18 | LENS, Lyme disease |
| Duncan's Story | Chapter 19 | Chelation for coronary artery disease |
| Melvin's Story | Chapter 19 | Chelation for coronary artery disease |
| Natalie's Story | Chapter 19 | Chelation for mercury toxicity |
| | | Cognitive dysfunction |
| Ingrid's Story | Chapter 21 | Ovarian cancer |
| | | Livingston vaccines |
| Larry's Story | Chapter 21 | MCS, LDA, methylation |
| Isaac's Story | Chapter 22 | Autism spectrum |
| | | Defeat Autism Now approaches |
| Nina's Story | Chapter 22 | ADHD/absence seizures (Petit Mal) |
| Calvin's Story | Chapter 24 | Mold toxicity, cognitive dysfunction, muscles spasms |

# Index

# About the Author

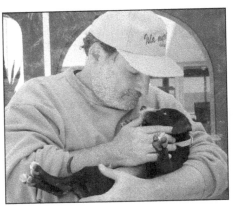

A graduate of the University of Chicago's Prizker School of Medicine, Dr. Neil Nathan has been practicing medicine for forty-one years. He is a board-certified family physician, and he has combined his knowledge of conventional medicine with his extensive background in holistic medicine and pain management in his efforts to provide diagnostic and therapeutic hope for those who have, unfortunately, "fallen through the medical cracks."

Dr. Nathan currently resides in Northern California with his wife, Cheryl, three dogs, and a cat. He is thoroughly enjoying the opportunity to savor their walks on the beaches and through the redwood forests on an almost daily basis.

He continues to practice medicine, do research, and teach both professionals and consumers. He and his colleagues, who provide the type of medical diagnosis and care described on these pages, can be reached for consultation or appointment at:

Gordon Medical Associates
3471 Regional Parkway
Santa Rosa, California 95403
Phone: 707-575-5180
FAX: 707-575-5509
E-mail: neil@gordonmedical.com